INTRODUCTION TO VETERINARY GENETICS

INTRODUCTION TO VETERINARY GENETICS

By

Dr. M. Prakash

Dept. of Zoology
M.M.H. Post Graduate College
Ghaziabad
(U.P.)

DISCOVERY PUBLISHING HOUSE PVT. LTD.
NEW DELHI-110 002

First Published-2009

ISBN 978-81-8356-430-4

Published by:

DISCOVERY PUBLISHING HOUSE PVT. LTD.
4831/24, Ansari Road, Prahlad Street,
Darya Ganj, New Delhi-110002 (India)
Phone: 23279245 • Fax: 91-11-23253475
E-mail: dphbooks@rediffmail.com
dphtemp@indiatimes.com
Website: www.discoverypublishinghouse.com

Printed at:
Sachin Printers

Preface

The present title "Introduction to Veterinary Genetics" has been designed for undergraduate, postgraduate students of Veterinary sciences having little or no background in Veterinary genetics. It is designed to serve as a general reference and textbook for a broad spectrum of applications. It is written to meet two objectives: (i) to provide those who need it with a sedimentary knowledge of chemistry and (ii) to present this knowledge within a framework of veterinary science, specially the genetics. It is designed to be simple, understandable, and interesting without being overly simplistic or misleading, it seeks to present the principles of genetics in ways so that even a reader with a minimal background in, or no particular aptitude for science and mathematics can master the material in it and apply it to a trade, profession or course of study.

To make the work more comprehensive and informative, the author has consulted many authoritative books, research journals, abstracts, monographs etc. He is grateful to all those great scholars whose work are cited or substantially reproduced.

There can be no claim to originality except in the manner of treatment and much of the information has been obtained from the books and scientific journals available in the different libraries.

The author expresses his thanks to his friends and colleagues whose continue inspirations have initiated him to bring out this book.

The author expresses his gratitude to Mr. Wasan and staff of M/s Discovery Publishing House Pvt. Ltd. for their whole hearted co-operation in the publication of this book.

In the mean time, the author will remain sincerely responsible for any shortcomings of the book and be grateful to the readers for their suggestions and constructive criticism for the continuous betterment of the book. He takes this opportunity to appeal to the readers to send their suggestions straightaway to his Publisher.

Author

Contents

1

INTRODUCTION

Although the basic principles underlying both plant and animal breeding are the same, their application to plants and animals has been different for several reasons. First, the numbers of individuals—the population sizes—which are available and can be handled conveniently in breeding and selection programmes are very much greater for plants than for animals. Second, the time that must elapse between one generation and another, the generation interval, is usually shorter in plants than in animals. Third, most individual plants can be fertilized by themselves or propagated vegetatively and so pure lines of plans can be obtained more easily than pure lines of animals.

These differences have had some important consequences for the methods and achievements of plants and animal breeders. For more than fifty years plant breeding has been done by genetics in national and commercial organizations who select, and organize the multiplication of, improved strains of plants for sale to farmers. The influences on animal improvement of organizations employing geneticists has been a more recent development; the role of the individual farmer-breeder has remained important. However, most farmer-breeders of livestock now work in cooperation with each other or with national or commercial organizations. This allows selection in animal populations which are often as large as those available to plant breeders.

Another consequence of the differences between plant and animal breeding is that the rat of change per year in performance which can be achieved by selection is greater for plants than for animals. The development of new techniques for stimulation earlier and more prolific reproduction is increasing the rate of change in both plant and animal breeding.

Domestication

Domestication is the process of developing strains of plants and animals which can be bred, handles and selected by man. Our domestic species and breeds of livestock originated, as did the cultivated varieties of plants, in different early centers of civilization and spread outward as the various civilizations extended throughout the world. Reindeer, dogs, sheep, goats, pigs, poultry and cattle were domesticated, probably in that order, over the period from 14000 to 5000 years ago. Much of the evidence for domestication comes from sites in northern Eurasia in the area between the rivers Euphrates and Tigris in Iraq and from Turkey, Syria and Jordan. From 5000 to 4000 years ago domesticated horses appeared in Asia and donkeys in north Africa. Domestication of the Ilama and guinea pig in occurred at that time. Attempts at domestication have not always been successful and it is known that efforts to domesticate the jackal and the hyena failed. New efforts to domesticate previously wild species such as red deer in Scotland and eland in Kenya are making progress.

The reasons why man domesticated animals are difficult to determine, through Zeuner (1963) has indicated a biological interpretation and Issac (1970) has suggested that domestication may be associated with the origins of religion. It is almost certain that domestication of species did not occur at a single site but was repeated at several sites

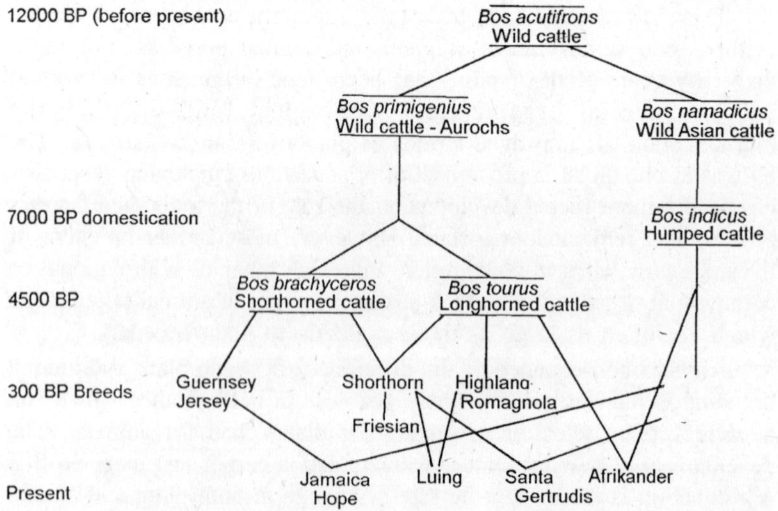

Fig. 1.1. A schematic development of modern cattle breeds by domesticaton from wild cattle.

at different times. In countries where a system of herdbooks is not in operation, such as parts of India and Africa, one finds types of animals associated with different tribes and regions. They have evolved partly by natural selection to suit local environmental conditions and partly by artificial selection. Many of these local types, or land races, have well marked fancy points such as colour and shape of horns but they also differ in productivity. Domestication has produced a considerable range of animal types within each species.

It is unfortunate that for most domesticated farm animals the wild populations from which they are descended have become extinct. Once the domesticated animals were found to be better than their wild relatives, man hunted and destroyed the wild populations so that they could not cross-breed with and spoil his improved stock.

Feral Animals

When an improved type of animal which has been reared and selected under good nutritional conditions is allowed to go 'wild' and again is subject to natural selection, with conditions of variable and often low planes of nutrition, its appearance tends to revert to that of its original wild ancestor. In New Zealand there are no native wild pigs, but when Captain Cook went there is 1772 he took some English domestic pigs and let them go wild. These 'reverted' pigs are today very similar to the wild boar in both conformation and composition; they are short in the body and long on the legs compared with the improved type. Moreover, the limb bones are thin and long as compared with those of the improved type just as the bones of wild sheep are thin as compared with those of sheep that have been improved for meat qualities.

Breeds and Conservation

During the eighteenth century and from among the variable land races, the early agricultural improves selected animals which form their appearance and from simple measures of performances suited the production systems and the market requirement of the time. In order to distinguish the selected groups the breeders standardized the external appearance of the animals. This process of selection led to the isolation of separate strains, many of which had different but desirable performance traits. Breeders with similar objectives and with similar looking stock then grouped together to form a breeding cooperative or breed society for the organizations of pedigree registrations, to ensure that the separate strains were maintained in reproductive isolation.

Most of today's breeds were established during the late eighteenth and nineteenth centuries. Since then there has been considerable selection within and between breeds, and breed substitution has been commonplace in many parts of the world. The widespread replacement of local breeds by the Friesian and Holstein for milk production is a good example.

Just as the wild ancestors of modern breeds, and many of the land races, of farm animals have become extinct through man's activities, so many breeds of livestock are being lost. Those breeds whose performance is not as good as other breeds at meeting contemporary economic needs become less popular, their numbers decline and very often they become extinct. Concern is now being expressed at this loss of valuable variation. The economic needs of the years ahead are not known and a breed which is unpopular today may carry characters which will be most valuable in the future. To safeguard the maintenance of variation in animals, conservation is being carried out for farm breeds of livestock just as it is for the wild species. Surgical ovum transfer has been used for breed substitution; the technique of deep freezing of semen and embryos offers a relatively cheap method for conservation of presently uneconomic breeds.

Livestock Improvement

Let us now consider the origin of the commercial characters of domestic animals. Under natural conditions wild animals are at the mercy of the environment, and in most places have abundance of food at one time of the year and little at another, consequently there is a regular seasonal variation in body weight. Very much the same conditions exist in the domestic animals of the less developed areas of the world and under some range conditions today. The limitation of food intake can inhibit the development of body conformation in cattle giving them almost the appearance of a different breed.

With the development of agriculture, however, conservation of food has made it possible to keep animals on a high plane of nutrition all the year round. Thus, by modifying some of the environmental conditions, it has been possible to breed and select for animals which reach puberty and lay down fat at younger ages, which it would have been impossible to do under the natural conditions of intermittent food supplies.

With the increase of fodder and cereal supplies has come the opportunity and desirability of breeding types of animals which will produce more, meat, milk, eggs and wool per animal or per unit of feed. A good nutritional environment is, in most cases, highly desirable for the selection of improved animals. The improved types of animals do not digest their feed more efficiently than the unimproved. The difference between them is mainly due to the way in which the nutrients are utilized by the body after absorption. For example, in order to make 45 kg liveweight gain the Poland-China breed of pig required only 189 kg of concentrate feed, whereas the first cross with the wild boar required 218 kg, and the backcross to the wild boar required 291 kg. An animal selected for meat or milk production therefore uses feedstuffs much more efficiently, in the sense that a higher proportion of the feed intake is utilized for production and a lower proportion is required for body maintenance. The distribution of the nutrient intake to the different parts of the body such as the skin, bones, muscles, fat and udder is determined by the nutrient intake level on the one hand and by the animal's genetic constitution on the other. Thus, if as a result of selection animals secrete more pituitary lactogenic hormone, or have mammary tissue which responds more sensitively to that hormone than their ancestors, the udder might be expected to be more developed and to utilize a higher proportion of the nutritional intake.

Breeding animals for commercial purposes such as meat, milk and eggs production is quite different from the creation of 'fancy' breeds. With the latter, the breeder is only concerned with aesthetic considerations. He takes some new mutation and make a breed of it, or includes the character in one or other of the existing breeds. By contrast, the breeder of horses for spread or draught, cattle for milk,

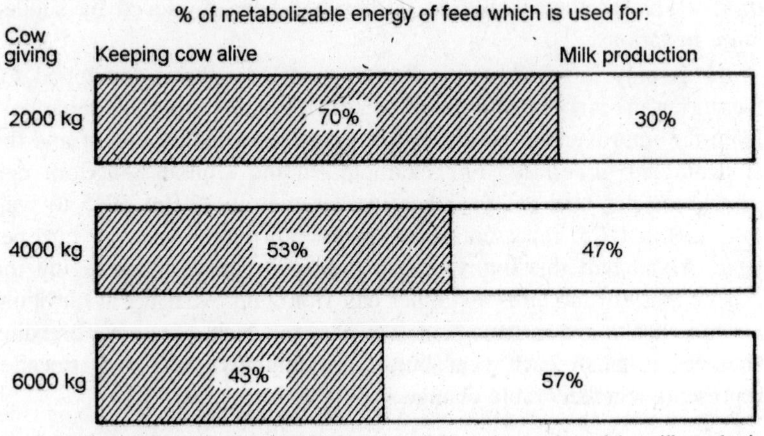

Fig. 1.2. Proportions of metabolizable energy used for maintenance and for milk production by cows with different annual yields.

or sheep for wool has a definite objective and directs the improvement of his animals. What this directed evolution means can be understood from the advice given to the prospective Merino flock master who 'must visualize the types of wishes to attain and the wool it is to grow. That "*dream sheep*" must be kept before his mind at all times'. As an example of what has been achieved by this method in Australia, the average fleece weight of adult sheep in New South Wales during 1881-5 was 2.3 kg while during 1956-9 it was 4.4 kg. However, this improvement is not due entirely to selection because during these years management also improved.

Another example of directional breeding is the Danish bacon pig. The present requirements for a good bacon pig are that it should have good feed conversion, length, this backfat, light shoulders and large hams. These were first specified by Danish producers and they set out to select for these characters under suitable and controlled environmental conditions in progeny-testing stations, with considerable successes. As the body composition of the pigs changed between 1924 and 1960, the feed conversion improved from 3.57 to 2.95. Again the improvements were not wholly due to selection because the management and environment in the testing stations were improved.

When an improve pig, such as the Danish Landrace, is crossed with the wild boar, from which it was originally derived, and the offsprings are mated back in each direction, there is a gradual transition from good to bad qualities in animals of different proportions of the genes of the two parent breeds. No qualities are completely dominant or recessive as they would be if they had been produced by sudden large mutations.

It is only in recent years that methods have been developed for measuring the amount of improvement achieved by selection separately from the improvement resulting from changes in management and the environment generally. For example, in the United Kingdom egg production per bird per year has increased from 120 in 1945 to well over 230 in 1975, representing an increase of over 3 eggs per bird per year. About half this improvement has been gained by changing the genetic merit of the birds and other half from improvements in nutrition, housing, health and management. The change which directional breeding achieves is small each year but it is cumulative and over decades represents a considerable change in production.

2

Mendelian Applications

Mechanisms of Inheritance

The observed or *phenotypic* characters in animals are the result of the genetic makeup or *genotype* of the animal and the environment in which it develops, lives and products. Characters are passed on from one generation to another by many genes, together forming the genotype, which are on the chromosomes within the cell nucleus. The chromosomes are formed by very long molecules of deoxyribonucleic acid (DNA) and each gene is a segment of one of these DNA molecules. Variations in the composition of the sections of DNA molecules are the gene differences which determine the development of the animal's characters throughout its life.

In the body cells of an animal, each of the chromosomes is duplicated. The number of chromosome pairs is the same for almost all individuals of a species but is different for different species. When the sex cells of animal are formed, a reduction, division, or *meiosis*, occurs and only one chromosome of each pair goes into the egg or the spermatozoon, so that only half the number of genes that are in the body cells of the animal go into the sex cells. When fertilization occurs the corresponding members of each chromosome pair, one from each parent, come together, and so the genes are duplicated in the body cells of the developing embryo. It is in this way that the characters from the two parents are transmitted to their offspring.

Occasionally during the formation of the sex cells the division of the chromosome pairs is not perfect. Also, during the division of the body cells, the replication of chromosome pairs is not always perfect. The results of these imperfections are cells with abnormal numbers of

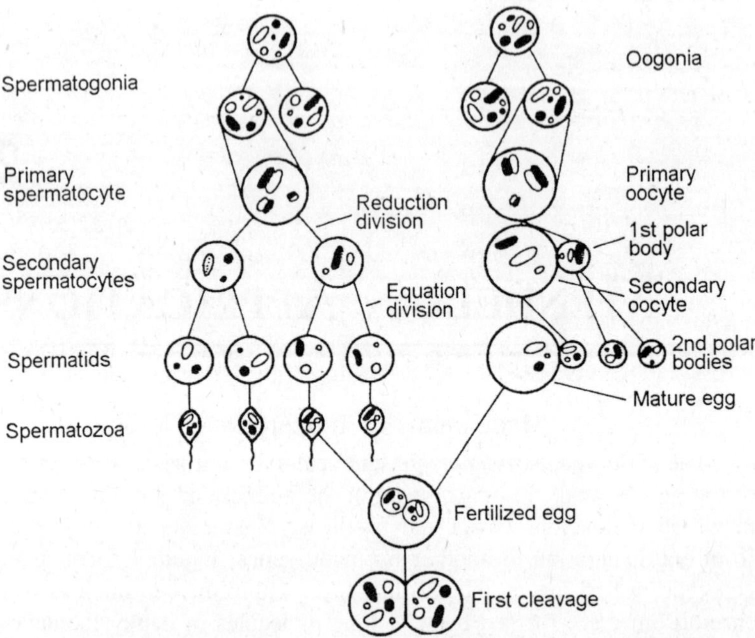

Fig. 2.1. The reduction division in the formation of sperms and eggs, showing how only one of each pair of chromosomes in the body cells of an animal pass to the germ cells.

chromosome for the species, sometimes too many and sometimes too few. Cells with abnormal chromosomes can survive but the individuals composed of such cells may be defective, so that they are mor prone to disease, they may not grow as quickly, or their productivity or reproduction may be poorer than that of normal individuals. Many chromosomes abnormalities which arise during the formation of sex cells lead to the very early death of the embryos which develop from such cells. Thus many chromosome abnormalities are eliminated before they can appear in adults.

Table 2.1. Normal chromosome number in farm animals; the numbers given include two sex chromosomes.

Horse	64	Goal	60
Donkey	62	Pig	38
Cattle	60	Chicken	78
Swamp buffalo	48	Mink	30
River buffalo	50	Dog	78
Sheep	54		

The special pair of chromosomes which determine sex are called the sex chromosomes. In mammals, the female has a pair of similar chromosomes called the X chromosomes and is termed the homogametic sex, while the male has one X chromosome and another quite different one called a Y chromosome, and is termed the heterogametic sex. It is clear that half the offspring of a female (XX) and a male (XY) will be XX, and therefore female, and half will be XY and therefore male. This accounts for the 50:50 sex ratio. In birds the sex chromosomes are designated by Z and W, the female is the heterogametic sex (ZW) and the male is the homogametic sex (ZZ).

The genes are located in definite places (*loci*), and the chromosomes maps may be made to show the distribution along the chromosome of the genes for particular characters. Characters which are controlled by genes on the same chromosome tend to be inherited together—they are said to be *linked*. However, at meiosis this linkage may be broken by a process of breaking and recombining of chromosomes, which involves *crossing over* between loci on sister chromosomes. This means that it is remarkably difficult to discover which genes lie on the same chromosome. The linkage groups have been found only by long and laborious breeding tests. In the larger farm animals few linkages have so far been found, and these involve blood group genes and genes concerned with body mechanisms for disease resistance. Other known genes appear to be transmitted independently—either they are on different chromosomes or they lie far apart on the same chromosome.

In an animal, *homozygous* for a particular character, both the controlling genes at the same position (locus) on each of a pair of chromosomes are exactly similar. When, however, the DNA constituting the gene at that locus undergoes a change of composition a *mutation* occurs, and when the sex cells of such an animal pair with the sex cells of a normal animal the paired genes (*alleles*) of the embryo are now different, alternative, forms of the gene, the normal and the mutant. Such *heterozygous* animals will not breed true, for at the next reduction division half the sex cells will have the normal gene and half will have the mutant form. If two such animals are mated together the chances are that two normals will unite once, two mutants once, and one normal and one mutant twice—giving an offspring ratio of one homozygous normal, two heterozygotes and one homozygous mutant.

For the most part these mutations are hidden (or *recessive*) in inheritance; that is, the heterozygous animal, which carries the mutant gene, is, in appearance, like the homozygous (or *dominant*) form. New

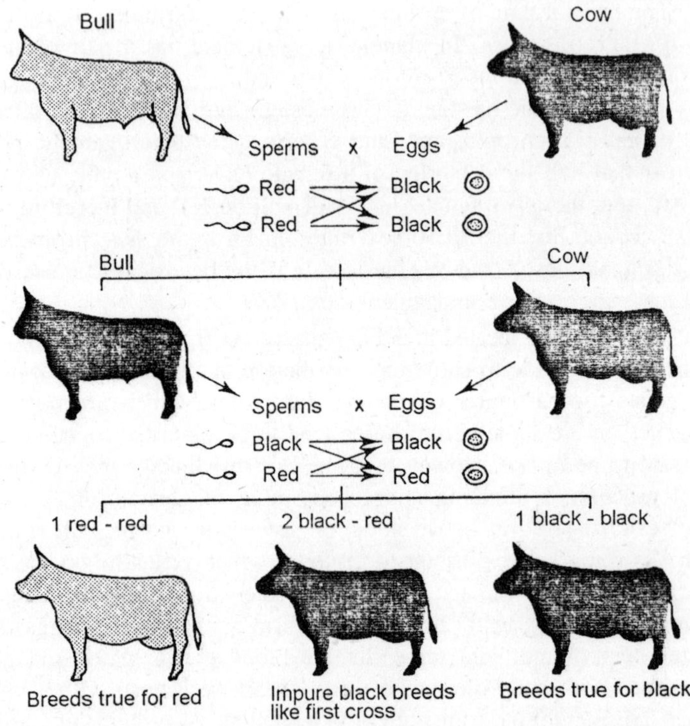

Fig. 2.2. Diagram to show how a pair of characters such as red and black colour in cattle are inherited; red is recessive to black.

mutants, which arise spontaneously with a very low incidence, are usually inferior to the normal alternative gene, and are eliminated from a population of animals by natural or artificial selection. Some of the mutations which appeared in the past have been used by breeders as a form of trademark to establish breeds.

Sex Linkage

It is thought that there are very few genes on the Y chromosome in mammals (or the W chromosome in birds). Therefore genes which are located on the X chromosome (Z in birds) will be linked or associated with sex and will be transmitted to the next generation in combination with sex. The fewer chromosomes the species has, and the larger is the X (or Z) chromosome, the more characters there will be associated with sex and inherited in a sex-linked way.

The practical application of sex-linkage occurs chiefly in poultry, in which it is a great convenience to be able to determine sex easily and early in life, so that pullets only can be reared when the chicks are wanted for egg production and the cockerels can be destroyed at hatching. The males of egg production strains of poultry are no use for broiler meat production. When the chicks are from strains to be used for broiler meat production the sexes can be identified and reared separately to improve growth rate and feed conversion.

The paired characters used for sex determination in poultry are early feathering as compared with late feathering, the down colours of silver as compared with gold, and whole coloured (dark heads) as compared with barred (light heads). When this sex-linkage in poultry was discovered, crosses between breeds were used for this purpose; such, for example, as discovered in crosses between two barred types (Plymouth Rock and Campine) that sex-linkage could be obtained within a breed breeding true for colours, such a breed (Cambar) was synthesized. More recently still it has been found that, provided the down colours of a bird are uniform, it is possible to make such a barred variety of any breed (Legbar, etc.) which will exhibit sex-linkage.

Auto-sex-linkage has not fulfilled its early promise. Birds must be bred primarily for production, so breeders cannot afford to restrict themselves to the barred breeds. Sexing is now done mostly by examination of external genitalia of the newly hatched chicks.

It seems unlikely that any commercial quality is wholly sex-linked, for commercial qualities are not simple mutant characters and do not depend on a single gene but on a large number of genes; it is unlikely that these genes are all situated on the sex chromosome.

Recombination of Characters

The method of recombination of characters has been use to a great extent in plant breeding; its application in animal breeding, however, has so far been very limited, not only because of the large numbers of individuals which must be eliminated in the process (and hence the cost), but also because of the time it takes to carry out. The following gives an example of recombination: we have a black-faced polled breed and a white-faced horned breed of sheep and wish to make a recombination, black horned or white polled, which will breed true. The first cross (F_1 generation) gives speckled-faced (intermediate) horned (dominant) animals; if these first crosses are now mated together to obtain the F_2 generation, this will contain a recombination of characters from which the combinations required can be picked.

This method of recombination is comparatively easy when both (as in the case in sheep quoted above) or one of the characters we wish to combine is of the simple mutant or Mendelian segregating type. Suppose, for example, it is desirable to make a polled Ayrshire having all the characters of the Ayrshire but being polled instead of horned. This milk characters of the Ayrshire are not of the simple

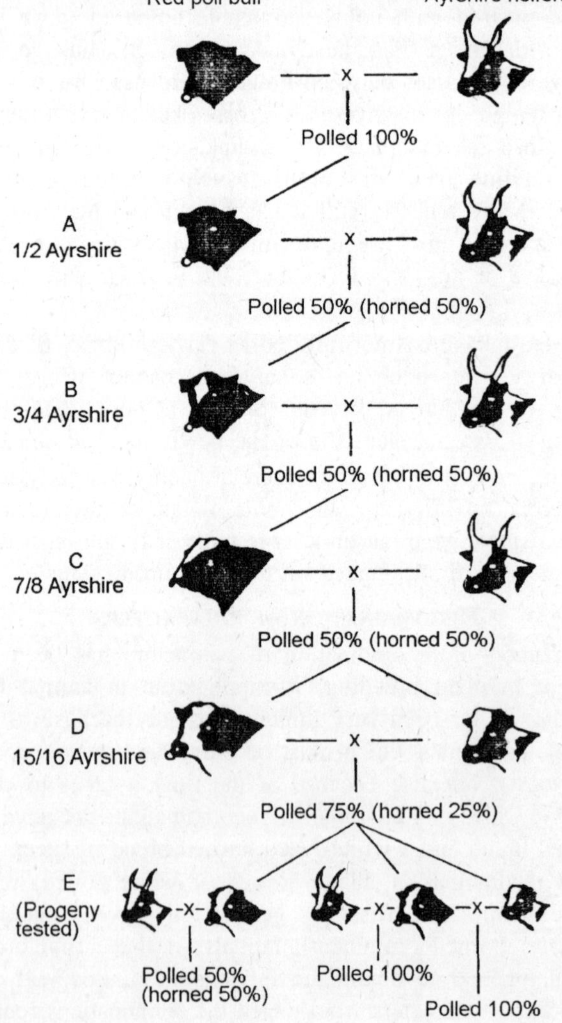

Fig. 2.3. Diagram showing how a character such as polled can be transferred from one breed to another.

Mendelian segregating type but show a blending from a inheritance. The horned and polled condition in cattle is, however, simple—polled being dominant to horned. If we mate a Red Poll but to an Ayrshire cow we obtain polled calves which will be heterozygous for the polled condition, but intermediate in body form. If we now mate a bull calf of this generation back to pure Ayrshire cows half his offspring will be polled, and all three-quarters Ayrshire in body type. We again pick out a polled bull calf from this generation and mate him to the pure Ayrshire as before, and the same thing happens again, except that the offspring will now be seven-eights Ayrshire in type. This is repeated until all traces of other than Ayrshire body characters have disappeared. At this stage the polled animals should be bred together and in this generation there will appear pure polled Ayrshire in the ratio of 1 in 4. To find out which are pure for the polled character the bulls should be mated with horned cows and those which fail to produce any horned offspring (progeny-tested bulls) should be kept for future breeding. If such progeny-tested bulls are used in successive generations the horned character will be bred out.

Some indication of whether a bull is likely to be, and breed, pure for the polled character can be obtained from an examination of his skull. If he has small scurs or bony lumps under the skin where the horns should be he is unlikely to breed true for the polled character. That is, in males the polled character is not completely dominant and heterozygous males may have lumps, small scurs or even small loose horns, depending on the breed. On the other hand, the polled character in most breeds is completely dominant in the female, although in a few breeds loose horns may occur. The heterozygous polled female therefore can only be detected by producing a horned or scurred male calf when mated with a pure horned or pure polled bull respectively. Polled strains have been, or are being, bred in many of the main horned beef and dairy breeds.

Blood Groups

The importance of blood groups for transfusions of blood in humans is well known. In man, horses and pigs, but not in cattle or sheep, when certain blood groups are present in the parents the newborn may suffer from a haemolytic disease which causes severe anaemia. In cattle (and also in sheep, horses and pigs) the blood groups are much more complicated that in man. These blood groups are inherited—no gene (allele) can be present in a calf unless it is present in one or both parents. Thus the blood groups can be used to check pedigrees and investigations have shown that in addition to deliberate falsification of pedigree, error can occur through a cow which is pregnant to one bull having a subsequent heat at which she is served by another bull. Another use for blood groups is in tracing the affinity between different breeds in all species of livestock.

In addition to differences in the red blood cells there are inherited variants of the blood serum proteins, of haemoglobin, and of the proteins in milk. Several investigations have indicated that there may be connections between some of these variants and productivity. For instance, cows carrying blood of one specific group have, on average, a higher milk-fat than those lacking it. Again, some specific types of serum proteins (transferrins) are associated with a higher milk yield. Some of these types can be assessed when the animal is comparatively young. It may not known whether the productive advantage associated with these particular proteins is due to the genes responsible for them, or to other genes closely linked on the same chromosome.

Coat Colour

The many varieties in coat colour in our domestic animals have all been derived by mutations from the normal wild-colour genes. In these, not only one but several mutations may occur, giving rise to a series (allelomorphic series) of different mutant genes, any of which may take their place as one of the pair at this locus of the chromosome. Thus, Adalsteinsson (1970) has shown that in Icelandic sheep 17 main colours of fleece, one white and 16 non-white, are distinguishable. There are three pigment types—tan, black and brown.

Tan (rust-red) pigment occurs only in the birthcoat of lambs, in kemp and outer coat fibres, and in fibres on hairy parts of the adult animal, whilst black or brown pigment may occur in all fibre types. White sheep either lack skin pigment completely or may have a little tan pigment. In non-white sheep, black or brown pigment may be present in addition to tan pigment. The inheritance of the tan pigment, which may occur in all the 17 main colours types, is not fully known. There are four colour patterns in non-white sheep; grey, badgerface, mouflon and grey mouflon, and are expressed whether the pigment is black or brown. In addition broken colour in non-white sheep can occur independently of pigment type and colour pattern. The 17 main colours are controlled by genes at three loci, A, B and S. At the A locus six alleles have been found. They are A_1, A_6, A_2, A_3, A_4 and A_5 which cause white, grey mouflon, grey, badgerface, mouflon and no pattern respectively. In this series inhibition of pigment is dominant to pigment production. At the B locus, the gene B_1 for black pigment is dominant to gene B_2 for brown pigment; at the S locus, the gene S_1 for unbroken colour is dominant to its allele S_2 for broken colour.

It is interesting to note that the A_1 allele has, in addition to the effect on coat colour, an adverse effect on fertility. This phenomenon of a single gene having multiple effects is called *pleiotropy*.

There may be two different genes giving rise to the same colour in a species. For example, in pigs, in most cases white is dominant to black, as, for example, in the Lincoln-Berkshire cross, but the white colour of the Mangalitza pig is recessive to black. Similarly in sheep, white wool is usually dominant to black, and black sheep are likely to occur in many white-woolled breeds; but in the Welsh breed there is a black which is dominant to white. This is the gene in the Black Welsh Mountain breed.

The white colour of albinos, which have pink eyes, is genetically quite distinct from the white colour of animals which have pigmented eyes. Physiologically an albino is an animal which lacks the capacity to form pigment, but it may contain the genes for any colour in its chromosomes. Albinism is recessive in inheritance, so when albinos are mated with coloured animals they produce young coloured according to the colour genes which they have inherited from their parents.

The coat patterns of animals behave in much the same way. A certain pattern may be present in an animal and yet not show itself until the colour genes are added, very much as the exposed film does not show up the picture until the developer is added. For example, the gene for striped coat is present in the wild boar, but in whit and in black pigs it never gets a chance to express itself. When, however, black and white breeds are crossed and a mixture of white and black hair (roan) is present, then the striped pattern appears in many animals.

In some breeds of animal, such as Himalayan rabbits and Siamese cats, the shade of colour which is produced by the gene depends on the skin temperature. The animals are born white and the general surface of the body where the skin temperature is high remains pale, but the extremities (nose, ears, feet and tail) become dark. Dark colours on the body can be produced experimentally by exposing areas to cold. Thus the effect the gene has on the character can be changed by altering the physiological conditions under which it acts. In those animals such as the mountain hare and ermine which change from coloured summer to white winter coats the mechanism is quite different. This is a photoperiodic effect; it is the change in the hours of daylight which induces the moulting of the dark coat in autumn, and of the white coat in spring.

Complete dominance of the normal over the mutation is not always found, and in many cases the heterozygous animal (containing both normal and mutant gene) takes on an intermediate form and so can be distinguished from the pure dominant. There is an example of this is the genes for red and white colour in Shorthorn cattle, in which the heterozygote is roan. Roans, having on the chromosome pair one gene for red and one for white, will never breed true; and if mate together will produce calves in the proportion of 1 red, 2 roans and 1 white. If one wishes to breed roans, the most certain way is to mate red cows with a white bull, or vice versa, for then all the calves will be roan.

Heterozygous Breeds

Before the mechanism of inheritance was fully understood frequent attempts were made to fix these intermediate heterozygous forms and make separate breeds of them. For example, in the Blue Albion breed of cattle the standard set up as the colour of the breed was like that of the roan Shorthorn, but with black in place of red. The consequence was, of course, that large numbers of black and of white animals, not eligible for registration, were produced, and no amount of selection will ever increase the percentage of blue roans. Another case that may be quoted is that of the Blue Andalusian fowl which is the heterozygous form of the black and the white colour genes, and so will never breed true. A third case of a breed being founded on an intermediate heterozygous form, caused inhibition of the growth in the length of the bones and produced a bulldog calf.

Such bulldog calves are not viable; they die and are aborted usually at about the 7th month. In the heterozygous condition, however, the gene for the bulldog calf produces merely a shortening of the legs. These animals had such an attractive appearance that breeders selected them and tried to breed them pure, with the result, however, that they continue to produce calves in the ratio of 1 long-legged, 2 short-legged and 1 bulldog. Bulldog calves can be avoided, however, by mating short-legged cows with a long-legged bull and vice versa, when calves will be produced in the ratio of 1 long-legged to 1 short-legged. This is an example of how a mutant character can, even if it is lethal in the homozygous condition, be carried on from generation to generation in the heterozygous condition. A somewhat similar bulldog mutation occurs in the Telemark breed in Norway.

Abnormalities

A large number of mutations have occurred, and are occurring, in our domestic animals, but practically all of the visible ones give rise to defective characters or fancy points. Some can greatly affect body size and conformation; for example in mice recessive genes are known which cause dwarfing and adiposity. At first sight some of them may appear to be of real economic value, for instance the double-muscled cattle have an increased proportion of muscle in the carcase, and correspondingly less fat and bone. Even this is of equivocal value, for the animals are unthrifty and infertile, (another instance of a pleiotropic gene) and so the character can only be carried on through the heterozygous form. However, the double-muscled bull can be cared for specially, and used for crossing on to normal cows to produce beef animals for slaughter only.

For the most part these mutations are the bane of the livestock breeder's life, for they give rise to degenerate and abnormal forms which detract from the efficiency of the animal in producing milk, meat, wool etc. The literature on animal genetics contains many descriptions of such mutant characters. A few will be quoted to illustrate the range of characters which may be affected and some of the generalizations which can be made about them.

Many mutants give rise to abnormal development of the embryo leading to foetal death or atrophy. In poultry they often cause death in the shell during incubation. These are the so-called lethal factors. Lists of lethal and sub-lethal characters in domestic animals have been published. Such lethal factors may be associated with some other character and so prevent its appearance in a pure (i.e. homozygous) form. One gene for yellow colour in mice is lethal in the pure form, while in the heterozygous conditions it causes extreme obesity. Likewise, dominant spotting in mice cause lethal anaemia when homozygous. The platinum gene in mink and silver fox is lethal in the homozygous condition. Dominant white is also probably lethal in horses—as in the Fredriksborg Stud of Danish horses.

While colour is often associated with other abnormalities. Hereditary deafness is common in blue-eyed white cats and in white dogs. While Shorthorn heifers often suffer from impaired development of uterus and vagina which renders them infertile. This is known as 'White heifer disease' and it also occurs in other white/roan coloured breeds such as the Belgian Blue. Another interesting example of this pleiotropic effect of a single gene is the connection between horenlessness and intersexuality in goats. Homozygous polled females are intersexual (often wrongly called *hermaphrodite*), or look like sterile males. Therefore it appears impossible to obtain a pure-breeding hornless breed of goats. Horns must be removed by chemical or electrical treatment of the horn buds. To produce normal polled goats (i.e. heterozygotes) one parent should be horned; half the offspring will be polled and half will be horned.

Mutations can be produced by treatment of the germ cell by radium or X-rays, which cause changes in the structure and the chemical composition of the genes. A very large proportion of such mutations, however, consist of gametic or early embryonic lethals, and thus lead to decreased fertility in the strain. Other mutations cause defects or abnormalities which make the animal less vigorous and less efficient commercially, and are of interest to the veterinarian in that they supply the explanation of cases he is often called on to treat. Examples of these are 'short-back' in cattle; atresia of the colon and sidebone in horses; earlessness and stiff joints in sheep; 'shakers' in goats; 'loco' in chicks; hydrocephalus, cleft palate, hernia, thickened legs, in turned nipples and imperforate anus in pigs; and cryptorchidism in goats, pigs, cattle and ships.

Many of these abnormalities are due to two or more pairs of genes acting together rather than to simple recessives. Complications in inheritance may also arise because only some of the animals homozygous for the gene concerned may show its effect (*penetrance* is incomplete). In other cases penetrance may be complete and all homozygous animals may be affected. In many case, also, *expressivity* is variable, i.e. the degree to which the abnormality shows itself in the individual varies greatly, although the gene which produces it is the same. This, for example, is so in a sex-linked lethal character (coloboma) which has been investigated in the chicken. In some embryos the abnormality may involve nearly all skeletal parts whereas in others it may be confined to a slight reduction of the upper beak. The probable explanation of these variations in the appearance of the character is that the defective gene interferes with the rate of cell division and with the rate of embryo development. The later stages of normal embryo development are dependent on normal completion of the earlier stages. Disruption of the early stages gives rise to variable abnormalities in the later stages. Thus, if the embryo is very slow in developing the abnormality is marked, whereas if the embryo is only slightly retarded the abnormality is slight.

A somewhat similar case of a recessive mutant gene giving rise to various degrees of an abnormality is that of the dropsical calf which occurs in the Ayrshire. Many of these have to be delivered by embryotomy and more are born dead than alive, although a few survive for a short time.

Similar mutants occurs in many different species; for example, the short dished face occurs not only in the bulldog, and in the Middle White pig, but has also appeared in cattle in the Argentine. 'Naked', or lack of hair, mutations have also occurred among normal animals of very different species—cattle and mice, for example. Other mutants such as dwarfing have been reported in the same species at different times and at different places.

Many of thee mutations, when they have not been too harmful, have been seized upon by breeders who have used them as the basis for new fancy breeds. In this way, for example, many of the queer shapes found in the different fancy breeds of dogs have been formed. As has already been mentioned, the production of 'fancy' breeds of animals is quite a different matter from the improvement of commercial qualities or natural evolution. As the vast majority of mutations are recessive in inheritance the production of 'fancy' breeds is relatively simple, for animals which show the character will breed true to it.

As will be appreciated from what has been said, many of these mutations are not so hardy as the original normal forms and this has probably given rise to the idea that the '*improved breeds*' are not so hardy and vigorous as the unimproved. This is true of many forms, such as the frizzle fowl, and the porcupine pigeon, but where the character affected is not such as to weaken the constitution of the animal, such, for example, as a colour change from grey to black hair a fancy breed may be equally as hardy as the normal dominant type.

Eliminating Unwanted Characters

We will now consider how we can purge our commercial breeds of livestock form the unwanted mutations which lower their efficiency for production, causing the appearance of a number of individuals tat are economically unprofitable.

Take, for example, the case of an inherited abnormality in pigs. As the unwanted characters are practically all recessive, if the young boars which are going to be the herd sires are mated with one or two sows which show the defective characters, any boar which is heterozygous will give offspring half of which will show the characters. Such boars can then be slaughtered. If, however, their offspring from affected sows are all normal then the boars can safely be used in the herd; and while such boars are used in the herd it is certain that the defect will never appear. It is better to start testing the males rather than the females on account of the larger number of offspring which they produce. Whereas the character is lethal the heterozygous female must be used; but in this case only 1 in 4 of the offspring of heterozygous males may be expected to show the character. This, however, is a counsel of perfection. A breeder would be better advised to get rid of all affected animals and their parents (which will be carriers) and to buy-in unrelated sires.

The prevention of the spread of unwanted characters throughout a breed is very important where males are used extensively, as in artificial insemination, in which one bull may sire sixty thousand calves a year. One way to guard against this is to mate the bull to be proved to 20 or more of his oldest daughters. If he carries any recessive defects, whether they be lethal, or of conformation or constitution, they will appear in the offspring. Sometimes if a defect becomes widespread in a breed it may be desirable to use special measures to reduce its frequency. In Galloway cattle a lethal defect known as tibial hemimelia syndrome has been found to affect between 1 and 2 per cent of purebred calves in Scotland. The defect is almost certainly caused by a recessive gene, and identification of heterozygous carriers is necessary to prevent them being used as parents of future purebred stock. The Galloway cattle society and the East of Scotland College of Agriculture have set up a special herd of cows which are all known to have given birth to a calf with tibial hemimelia and therefore are heterozygotes. The purpose of the herd is to test-mate bulls which might be used widely in the breed. Each bull is mated to produce a minimum of ten calves, which will permit the detection of at least 94 percent of heterozygous bulls. The defect is obvious in 90 days old fetuses, so in order to test more bulls in the special herd the cows are deliberately aborted at 90 days by prostaglandin treatment. This allows two test fetuses per cow per year, instead of less than one if the fetuses were allowed to continue for a full gestation period. In practice an artificial insemination sire carrying a recessive defect usually shows up without special testing. There are enough carriers among the general female population to which he is mated; and one in four of their offspring will be abnormal if the bull is heterozygous for the same gene.

3

Quantitative Genetics and its Application

Unit and Multiple-factor Characters

Up to this point those characters which are dependent on one gene only have been mainly considered. Unfortunately none of the commercial characters, such as body composition, growth rate, milk and butterfat yield, egg production, fleece weight, come under this heading. While unit factors (single genes) give rise to most of the defects and fancy points, all the commercial qualities investigated have been shown to be due to more than one gene; thee are called multiple-factor characters.

Commercial qualities are in the main quantitative rather than qualitative and so cannot be measured as a fixed point, but must always be measured as a frequency-distribution curve about a mean. For example, although two breeds of cattle differing substantially in their mean butterfat percentages can be obtained, it is impossible to obtain a breed in which there is no variability in butterfat percentage. This defines it is a quantitative character which varies in amount not only with the genetic constitution but also with the physiological conditions and physical environment of the animal. When two breeds differing materially in their butterfat percentage are crossed together, the butterfat percentages of the resultant offspring fall on a distribution curve with a mean intermediate between that of the two parent breeds. When a second generation is raised by back crossing the first to the two parent breeds, the character is again intermediate, that is, there

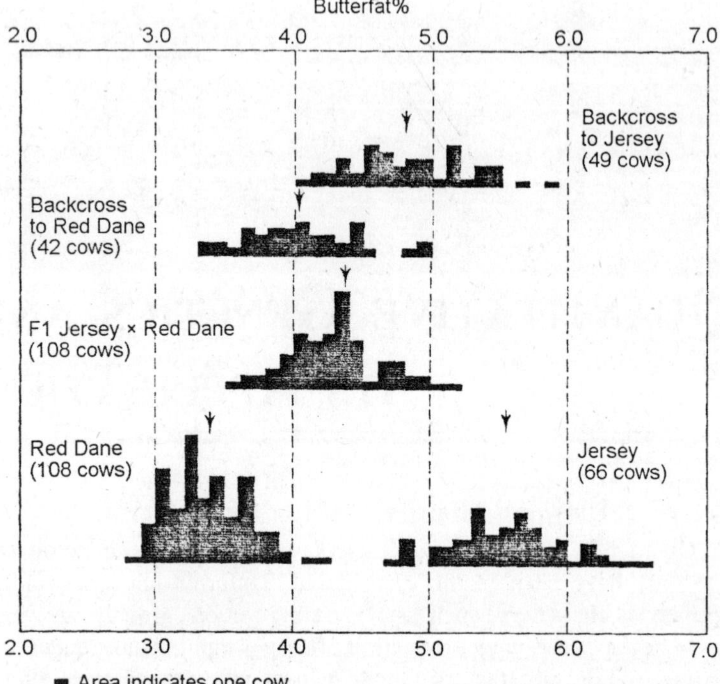

Fig. 3.1. Inheritance of butterfat percentage in crosses and back crosses between Red Danish and Jersey cattle. Arrow indicates average for each group.

is no dominance or recessiveness, but the commercial character has a blending form of inheritance. This is the usual way in which commercial characters like milk production are inherited. Physical characters, too, such as size, weight and body dimensions, are inherited in the same way.

Genotype and Environment

The development of all these characters of economic importance is dependent on the environment in which the animal is kept and reared. Changes in performance on farms are usually a combination of changes in environment and changes in the genetic quality of the animals. For example, the increase in the average milk yield for recorded cows in England and Wales during the past thirty years is the result of improvements in nutrition, husbandry, disease control and the genotype of the cows. Some environmental factors such as age, dry period before calving and frequency of milking (2 or 3 times daily) affect the yield of milk given by a cow, and correction factors

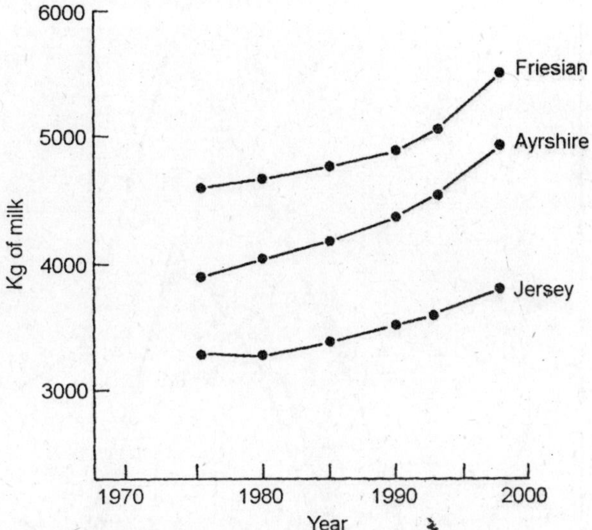

Fig. 3.2. Changes in herd average cow lactation yields; recorded herds in England and Wales, yields uncorrected for differences in milk quality.

have been calculated to correct yield for these factors, so as to obtain a better comparison between individuals differing in these respects.

Only by adopting special techniques or by setting up special tests is it possible to demonstrate the extent to which differences between individuals and breeds are the result of environment or genotype. For example, it is possible to breed populations of animals which remain of constant genetic quality over many generations. These 'control' populations can be used to measure differences in performance caused by changes in the environment of which the farmer may otherwise be unaware.

The variation between animals refers to animals reared under the same conditions and fed in the same way. Even within a herd where each cow is given the same treatment of equal opportunity, where disease is absent and age of calving is identical, there still remains environmental differences between cows which often have more influence on the yield than do the genetic ones. It is these largely intangible effects within a herd to which the geneticist is referring when the speaks of '*environmental variation*'. And it is the combination of the environmental effects and the effect of many genes, each with a small effect (multiple factors), which causes the variation in breed type. The difference between the average of the two breeds and between the breed crosses, on the other hand, is entirely genetic.

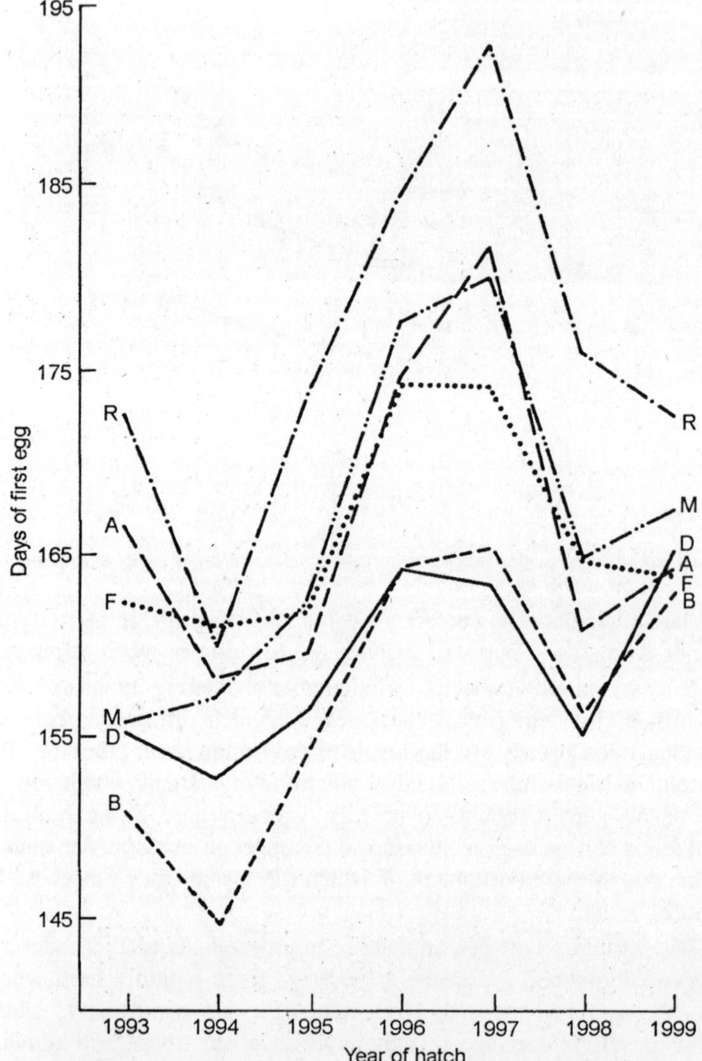

Fig. 3.3. Variation in age of sexual maturity (ddys to first egg) of six poultry strains, each bred to keep the same genetic composition from generation to generation.

Heritability

Some characters of an animal are inherited strongly while in others the intensity of inheritance is much lower because their development in the animal is more dependent on environmental conditions. The intensity of inheritance can be measured as the proportion of the superiority of the parents (over the herd or population mean) which is passed on to the next generation. This is called the '*heritability*' of a character. The values of heritability are specific to the population on which they are measured. There may be substantial differences of heritability for the same character between populations with different breeding histories, or kept in different environments.

Table 3.1. Heritability of characters in beef cattle.

Character	*Preferred values of heritability Per cent*	*Range of observed values*	*Degree of heritability*
Calving interval	5	2–20	low
Service period	5	3–13	low
Twinning	3	–	low
Gestation length	40	0-83	medium
Birth weight	38	0-100	medium
Pre-weaning growth rate (up to 6-8 months)	27	0-68	low-medium
Weaning weight	30	0-100	medium
Daily gain in feedlot	52	0-100	medium-high
Final weight	70	12-100	high
Feed intake	44	35-76	medium
Feed conversion	36	17-99	medium
Carcase fatness-fat thickness over longissimus dorsi	50	24-74	medium
Longissimus dorsi area	40	3-100	medium

The heritability of characters tends to be lower the more closely they are associated with reproduction. Thus in beef cattle the heritability of calving interval is about 5 percent, of weaning weight is about 30 percent and of carcass fatness about 50 per cent. This is a useful general guide to the level of heritability for all species.

It appears that the heritability of a character, and so the accuracy with which selection can be made, is greater when the environmental conditions are standardized, for then the differences in the expression of the character between individuals are more the result of heredity and less the result of environment.

The difference in the heritability of different characters, due to the degree to which they are dependent for their development on environmental conditions, is illustrated in identical twins in cattle, which being derived from one egg, have the same genetic constitution.

In such characters as colour, hair whorls and shape of horns, twins are very similar to each other because these characters are little affected by the environment. When, however, such twins are reared on very different planes of nutrition, the late-developing parts of the body can show considerable differences. Bonnier et al. (1948) found that the level of nutrition which was necessary to bring out the full genetical potential varied for different characters. The ceiling levels followed the growth gradients in that the head and forequarters were fully developed at a lower level of nutrition than that needed for full development of thé hindquarters. Milk yield needed a lower level than complete body form.

Incidentally, identical twins can be used to measure the effect of nutrition, and of environment generally, independently of genetic influences. For example, using 120 pairs of twins and by placing one twin of each pair in a high-yielding dairy herd and the other in a low-yielding one, it has been demonstrated that the major part of the differences in milk and fat yield between the two groups of herds are due to the methods of feeding and management rather than to heredity. Though identical twins have been used in the past to measure heritability, the values obtained in this way are usually substantially too large because of the large common maternal effects.

Selection

In any part of the body where variability exists, the selection and breeding together of the variant animals lead to changes in the character concerned. Thus, for example, while most sheep have only 2 nipples, some are occasionally found with 3 or even 4, and by selecting and breeding together such multi-nippled sheep it has been found possible to obtain ewes with 6 functional nipples. Similarly, while the pig has usually only 14 thoracic vertebrae and ribs, individuals occur in which the number is 15, 16 or even 17, and it is found that on the whole such animals have longer bodies. By breeding together animals showing this variation, strains with large numbers of ribs may be produced. The higher the heritability of a character the more rapid the improvement expected from selection. A good example of what can be achieved has been shown by Hetzer and Harvey who, starting from a single pig population, selected one strain with more backfat and another with less backfat in each of two breeds. After 10 generations of selection in Durocs the high strain had an average of over 5 cm of backfat thickness whereas the low strain had less than 3 cm. In Yorkshires, eight generations of selection resulted in a difference of over 1 cm backfat thickness. Much has been learnt about selection methods by experiments on laboratory animals such as the fruit fly (*Drosophila*) and mice.

One of the first and most different aspects of selection is the choice of objectives. Not only is it necessary to select animals on the basis of characters which can be easily measured early in life and which are the main determinants of profit form the animal, but it also is necessary to have regard for the future market requirements perhaps 5-20 years hence. The improved animals produced by selection will be used in a future economic setting rather than the present one.

Selection is only possible under conditions in which a character is expressed. This applies for instance to milk production. Food intake is used for the maintenance of the body first, and only the surplus is used for production; consequently where food supplies are limited the genetic capabilities of the animal for milk production are not demonstrated and proper selection cannot be made. From this it has been concluded that when we wish to direct the improvement of an animal in any respect we should keep the population under selection in an environment which allows full expression of the character in question and rigorously select and breed from those individuals which show the character to the fullest extent. This is not necessarily so. For milk yield, for instance, bulls give a similar progeny test result whether tested in a poor environment (low-yielding herd) or a good one (high-yielding herd). The advantage of testing in a good environment is that the heritability is usually higher and therefore fewer daughters are needed for an accurate progeny test.

Experiments on body size in mice have given equivocal results. Those by Falconer (1960) indicate that, for growth rate, it is better to select animals on a low plane of nutritional. Dalton (1967), on the other hand, got the same results whether he selected animals on a full diet or on one diluted with cellulose.

In view of this discrepancy between results, and of the differences between species and between characters, it is not safe to generalize either for or against selecting under optimal environmental conditions. However, there are records from most farm animals to show that the rank order of performance for breeds and families is not the same for different environments. Breeds have been developed to suit particular farming requirements. Therefore it is probably safest to select breeding animals under conditions which are as close as possible to those under which their progeny are to be exploited commercially.

Performance Testing

In order to select the best parents for breeding, the animals available must be compared under standard conditions. Thus in order to compare animals from different herds, and therefore different environments, they must be brought together under the same conditions of feeding and management. Such as arrangement is called a '*performance test*'. Its greatest use is for selecting males, and it can be used only for characters such as growth rate and feed-conversion efficiency which can be measured on a sire without slaughtering him. It is thus very important for evaluating beef bulls. Within the development of ultrasonic methods of back fat measurement in pigs, performance test of boars is tending to replace progeny testing.

Performance testing is measuring the characters in the sire himself, as contrasted to progeny testing which measures the characters in his offspring. When a character is fairly strongly inherited and where provision is made for a constant environment (including nutrition and management) the performance testing of males will give quicker, although less accurate, results than progeny testing; it will at any rate eliminate some males before progeny testing.

Progeny Testing

The progeny test is the measurement of the genetic value of the animal in question by the production records of its offspring. Since a male produces during his lifetime many more offspring than a female, the progeny test is applied much more widely to males than to females. The progeny test is of the highest importance for those products, such as milk and eggs, which the male does not produce himself, but only transmits the capabilities of producing to his female offspring.

Progeny testing of sires is only justifiable if it increases the rate of genetic improvement per year compared with other methods of selection. It does so if the character under selection is not measurable in adult animals of both sexes, if its heritability is low, if the breeding unit is large, and if the increase in the generation interval, which is inevitable with progeny testing, is not disproportionately large. The first three of these criteria apply to milk yield in dairy cattle bred by artificial insemination; the increase in the generation interval is counterbalanced by the advantages of progeny testing. This is therefore the best method to use in selection for milk yield. In breeding for egg production in poultry, progeny testing increases the generation interval by 100 per cent; family selection therefore turns out to be the best method. Family selection is similar in practice to progeny testing except that the individuals chosen as parents of the next generation are the animals of the best families on test and not their parents as would be the case in progeny testing.

The generation internal tends to be shorter for family selection than for progeny testing, but the number of superior animals which can be produced may be less. In pig breeding a further consideration is important. Here special testing facilities are necessary, which if used for sires rather than for progeny very much increases the number of sires which can be tested and therefore also increases the selection intensity among sires. With the development of methods for estimating the fatness of live pigs, the trend is to use more of the limited facilities of the test station for performance testing and less for progeny testing.

Maternal Effect

One aspect of the environment which has a profound effect on some characters is the prenatal environmental provided by the mother. Body size is particularly affected. When reciprocal crosses are made between the large Shire horse and the small Shetland pony, the size of the offspring in each case is considerably affected by the size of the dam. Similarly the mule with the horse as dam is a larger animal than the reciprocal cross, the hinny with the donkey as dam. This maternal effect on size is made use of in mule breeding, where the most desirable mules are bred by first crossing the large Percheron mare with the smaller but more active and spirited Thoroughbred stallion; the large active mare so produced is mated with a donkey stallion to introduce the character of heat resistance; thus large, active, heat-resting mules are obtained. Maternal effects on size have also been shown in reciprocal South Devon × Dexter cattle crosses. Maternal effect on size in rabbits has been strikingly demonstrated by O. Venge, who transplanted the fertilized eggs of a small breed of rabbit into a doe of a large breed and the eggs of a large breed into a doe of a small one.

Maternal effects are also shown in Border Leicester × Welsh sheep crosses and in transplanted ova. These maternal effects last for some considerable time after birth in both sheep and cattle. In horses they persist up to adult life because length growth below the knee and hock is completed at birth. In other species where the proportional length of the lower limbs is not so well developed at birth there is scope, according to the state of its development at birth, for the growth to be made up by good feeding.

ADAPTATION TO ENVIRONMENT

In addition to selecting for productivity under ideal conditions, the breeder of livestock has also to breed for constitution, or the power to live and thrive under the conditions in which the animal is kept. Under natural conditions selection for this is by elimination of the unfit. This is one of the reasons for the occurrence throughout the world of so many local breeds of sheep, for the conditions under which sheep are kept come nearer to natural conditions than those for most other varieties of our livestock.

Let us now consider some exampled of this. While European breeds of dairy cattle have a constitution eminently suitable for life in temperate climates, when they are transported to hot and humid tropical climates it is found that their tolerance of heat is limited. Their body temperature and rate of respiration go up and their appetite declines. As a result of this poor heat tolerance, much more time is spent lying

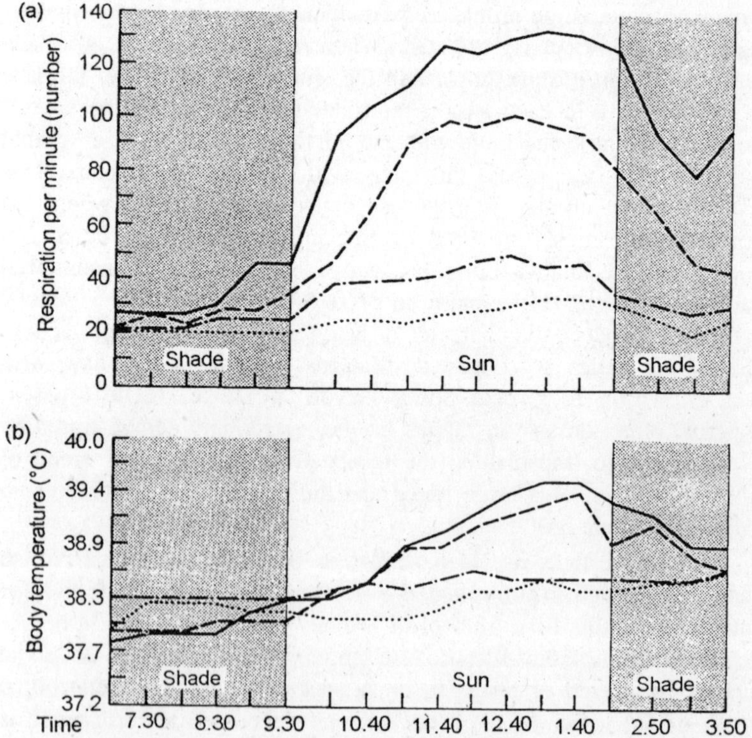

Fig. 3.4. Respiration rate (a) and body temperature (b) of cattle removed from the shade and exposed to strong sunlight on a summer day.

in the shade rather than grazing. Under these conditions of low food intake or utilization, growth is retarded, the age of puberty is delayed and milk yields decline; in fact in a few generations the breed degenerates. In addition, tropical climates exert much of their adverse effect on production indirectly by lowering the quantity and quality of pasture and fodder crops available. Zebu cattle, however, which have developed in the tropics, have a constitution suited to their surroundings (good temperature regulation in hot humid climates and ability to thrive on low-quality fodders) but are poorly developed in the milk-secreting tissues of the mammary glands. When crosses are made between European and Zebu cattle under humid tropical conditions the offspring grow better and yield more milk than either parent because from the one they receive udder development, while from the other they receive the constitution which enables the body to supply to the udder the nutrients required for milk production.

The severity of the climatic conditions will naturally determine the relative proportions of blood of each which are required to give the optimum results; lifetime yields are, of course, a better criterion than maximum lactation yields. The Indian Army Dairy Farms obtained such a striking improvement by making crosses of native cows with imported Ayrshire and Friesian bulls that they continued the introduction of European blood. There came a time, however, when the percentage of European blood became too high, and then production fell instead of increasing. By introducing into this 'degenerate' stock more Zebu blood and so a constitution suited to the tropics, production is increased. In beef cattle, experiments along these lines have taken place in Queensland, Australia, and also in the southern states of the U.S.A. In both countries the first cross between Zebu and British breeds is strikingly superior to either pure breed. In Texas a new breed, the Santa Gertrudis, has been produced by combining the beef qualities of the Shorthorn (five-eighths) and the heat tolerance of the Zebu (three-eights).

Some characters in animals which may be an advantage in one climate may be a great disadvantage in another. For example, the thick winter coat in certain breeds of cattle holds a blanket of warm air round the skin and this, unless exposed to wind, insulates the body from cold. When such breeds are taken into tropical climates, however, many individuals fail to got into a short summer coat and so fail to regulate body temperature and do not thrive. The reason why the moult of the winter coat of many British breeds fails to occur in the tropics

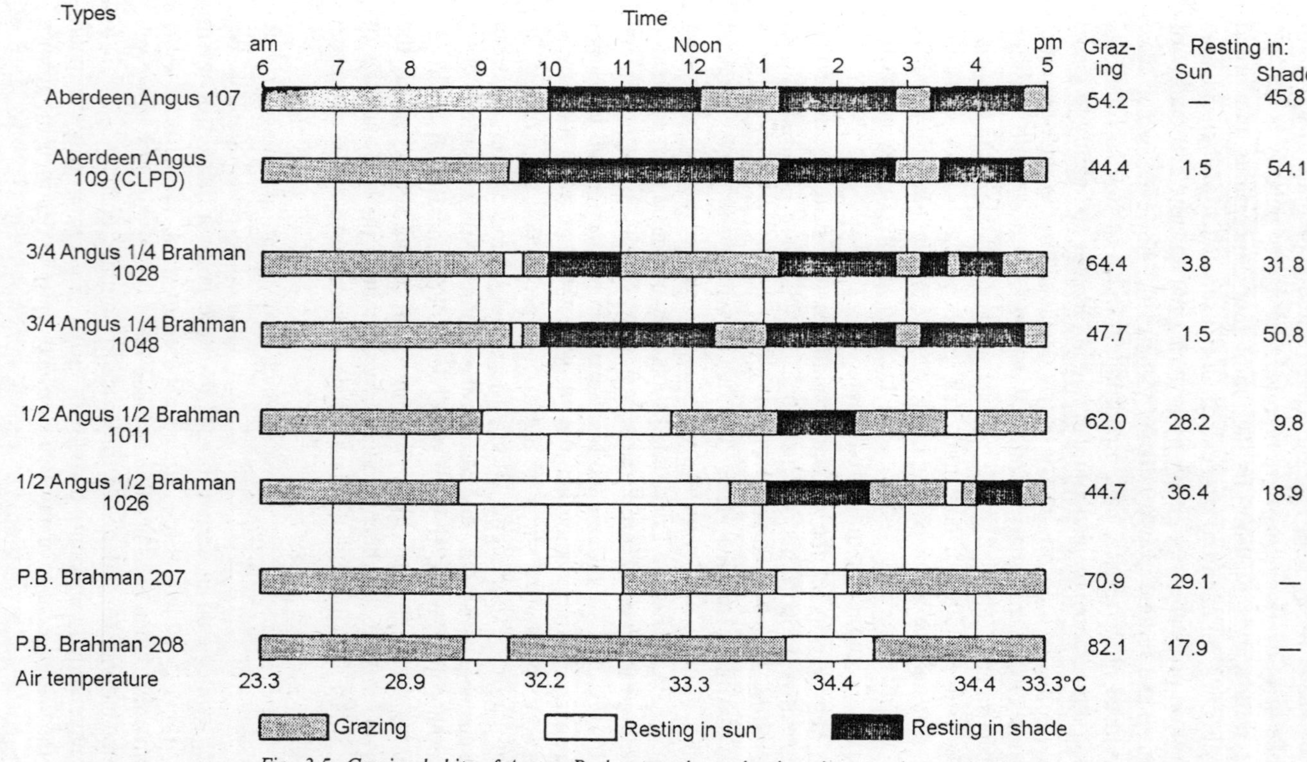

Fig. 3.5. Grazing habits of Angus, Brahman and crossbred cattle on a clear and calm day.

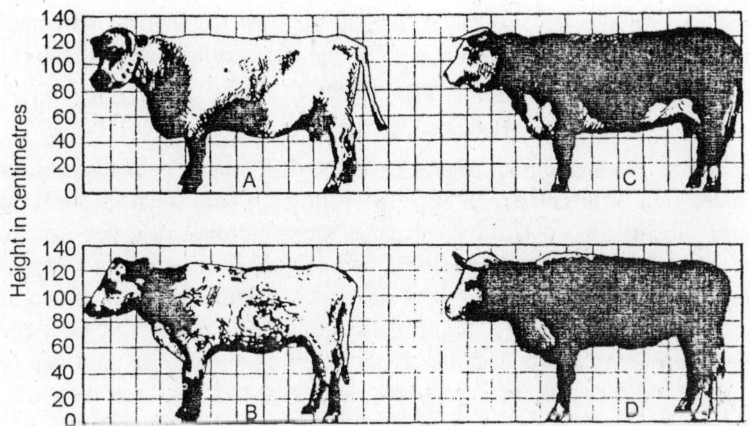

Fig. 3.6. Changes in type due to being grown under adverse high-temperature conditions. Shorthorn cow (A) under optimum conditions and (B) under high-temperature conditions. Hereford cow (C) under optimum conditions and (D) under high-temperature conditions.

is that it is controlled by photoperiod. High temperatures also affect pregnant mothers in breeds that are not heat-tolerant, so that calves and lambs born after a very hot period are smaller than normal. It has been shown that one of the reasons why Zebu breeds are more heat-tolerant than British breeds is that they sweat more. Selection for heat-tolerant characters in British breeds of cattle to suit them for the tropics is now taking place in Queensland. Heat tolerance is measured by the rise in body temperature when the air temperature is raised, or after exercise. Such tests show that, of European breeds so far tested, the Jersey is one of the best in this respect. The heat-regulating powers are not so well developed in the young animal as in the old one, and so selection for heat tolerance is best carried out in the calf stage.

Another example of the poorer heat-regulating powers of the young animal is seen in the pig, where owing to lack of coat covering the young animal suffers much from cold and draughts and so fails to grow properly, the critical temperature being 15.5°C for old pigs but 24°C for young pigs. In pigs the subcutaneous layer of fat forms an insulator against heat loss. In newborn pigs there is little subcutaneous fat so that death from cold are often considerable particularly where insufficient milk is available during the first few hours after birth.

The effects of climate on the animal's performance are very great and play an important part in the evolution and selection of domestic animals. The climate and environmental conditions of an area playa large part in the success of selection for any particular character. They also form one of the causes for the regionalization of different types of commercial livestock production.

Disease Resistance

Among small animals many cases of differences in susceptibility to disease in different strains have been found. (This situation must be sharply distinguished from the case of constitutional diseases caused by mutations and hence behaving s unit factors in inheritance). In the sphere of infectious or contagious diseases, certain strains of mice are highly resistant and others highly susceptible to leukaemia, mammary cancer, pseudorabies and mouse typhoid. In all such cases care has to be taken to distinguish between true genetic resistance and the immunity

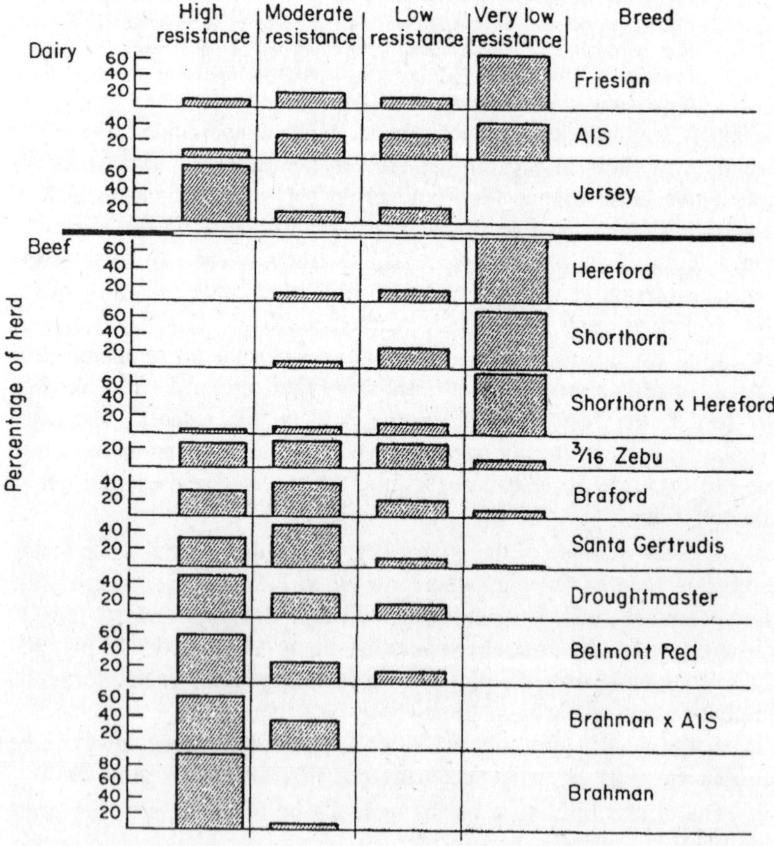

Fig. 3.7. Frequency distribution of resistance to cattle tick in heifer herds of vaious breeds.

which is acquired by the offspring *in utero* or through the mammary secretions of the parent.

There is good evidence that susceptibility to some diseases in cattle is inherited, for example mastitis and Johne's disease, but the heritability is low. In our larger farm animals the process of obtaining resistant strains by selection in an environment of disease would take too long and would be far too expensive to warrant consideration. Furthermore, the reproduction rate in bacteria is high, and they can produce new virulent strains by mutation quicker than immune strains can be produced in domestic animals. African and Asian Zebu cattle have not developed immunity to prevailing disease such as rinderpest and trypanosomiasis. They seem to be less susceptible to tick infestation than European cattle and more tolerant of the tick-borne fevers, but they still need natural infection as calves to acquire immunity as adults. Some African humpless cattle such as the West African Dwarf Shorthorn and the N'Dama appear to be tolerant of trypanosomiasis.

A special and interesting case is afforded by cancer of the eye which occurs in white-faced European cattle (chiefly Herefords) in the tropics. Investigations in Texas have shown that it strongly inherited and furthermore that cancer of the eyelid (but not of the eyeball) occurs only on unpigmented eyelids. The disease can thus be reduced by using 'cherry-eye' Herefords.

4

Breeding, Inbreeding and Crossbreeding

In the past the showyard had played a large part in moulding our breeds of farm animals. Criticism of this method have been made on the basis that selection has tended to follow appearance rather than commercial qualities. However, the changes in body conformation and composition, in wool quality and yield, and in milk let-down and yield which were effected by the methods of breeders in the 18th and 19th centuries, should not be underestimated. Though these agricultural improvers, such as Bakewell and the Collings brothers in the U.K., kept few records and used fairly simple selection methods there is no doubting the beneficial effect they had on the performance of farm livestock.During the last thirty years there have been substantial developments in the selection methods used, in the size of populations available for selection and in the ease of collecting, storing and analysing large numbers of performance records. The appearance of an animal on the farm or in a showyard is still an important element in determining whether it will be chosen to be a parent of the next generation. However, its performance and that of its close relations for characters of commercial significance are now of overriding importance in the selection process. A high performing animal will be used as a parent if it also has a good appearance but a poor performing animal will be culled however good its appearance.

Selection Objectives

The first thing to do when starting a selection programme is to decide objectives (characters to be selected) and this can be much more difficult than is often supposed. It is necessary to define accurately those characters which are commercially important now and those which will be important to 15 years hence, for the animals from the selection programme will not have much effect on commercial production until then. Having defined characters in this way, difficulties arise because there are usually too many of them for selection to be effective and some of them may not be capable of direct measurement without considerable expense or without killing the animal. These problems can be illustrated by reference to beef cattle. Table 4.1 shows some characters which might be subjected to improvement by selection. This list exemplifies some of the difficulties in choosing selection objectives. Growth rate can be measured easily, relatively accurately and cheaply. Feed conversion is more difficult. The feed intake of individual animals can only be obtained by recourse to individual penning or to the use of electronically controlled gates, which allow each animal access to its own individual feed trough even though the animals are housed in groups. Both methods are unlike conditions found on commercial units, so that feed intake measurements obtained under test conditions may be unrepresentative of those on farms. Carcase quality measurements can be obtained effectively only by slaughtering the animal, though new techniques for measuring carcases in live animals will reduce considerably the number which have to be slaughtered to measure carcase characters. Thus it is necessary to store semen from potential breeding males before slaughter, or to rely on the records of carcase quality of relatives, to be able to select for these carcase characters. The cost of measuring carcase traits is high. Resistance to disease is very difficult to select for because of the problems associated with offering an equal and realistic field challenge to each animal. Behaviour characters are still largely described in qualitative terms which do not make selection easy.

Table 4.1. Characters which might be included in selection objectives for improving cattle for beef.

Growth rate	Carcase quality
Feed consumption	killing out percentage
Feed conversion	learn percentage
Resistance to disease	fat percentage
Behaviour	meat colour
docility	meat tenderness
	keeping quality
	eye muscle area

This example of choosing character for selection is not atypical and it can be appreciated why selection in beef cattle has been concerned largely with growth rate and appearance. It is well to remember that the more characters included for selection the less the likely progress for each of them.

Selection to Suit Farm Environments

As part of planning a selection programme it is necessary to determine the possible range of farm production systems in which the animals will be used, and whether different selection schemes will be needed to breed specializes strains for each system. Selection will usually be under the system giving maximum expression to the character being selected. In general, strains of livestock are extremely adaptable to a range of conditions. Only if extreme environments or very different market circumstances are considered is it found necessary to contemplate more than one selection programme. Generally it is simpler and more profitable to eliminate the extreme of environment by altering the production system than to multiply the number of selection programmes.

Structure of Animal Breeding Programmes

Until about 1950, most animal breeding was the responsibility of individual herd owners. However, the more important programmes are now the responsibility of several other types of organization. These include government organizations, breeder cooperatives and breeding companies. The latter having started to select one animal species, mainly poultry (or even plants), have in several cases diversified to reed several species. It is interesting to discuss the reasons for these developments. In the first place a very large population is not essential for genetic progress, so that there is nothing to deter one individual herd owner from continuing a constructive breeding programme with the animals at his disposal. However, the cost of testing animals, and of culling animals in order to apply so worthwhile selection pressure, is high in relation to the cost of production. Also there is no double that the larger the population under selection the greater the chance of success. The cost of the programme has to be more than recopied if the breeder is to remain in business. It maybe several years between the start of the selection programme and the time when the benefits in terms of improved animal performance can be recouped by the breeder, by the sale of stock to commercial producers. The breeder has to carry the cost for this period. The more progeny produced from improved stock, the lower the cost of the programme as a charge on each animal produced. This multiplication, marketing, and indeed organization, play extremely important roles in the financial success and long term viability of breeding programme. These programmes are dependent on fast data processing equipment, on technical advice and on continuing access to new genetic developments, all expensive facilities. However, since the principles are similar irrespective of the species, it is not difficult to run simultaneously several breeding schemes, for different species, using the same technical resources. Savings in marketing costs can also be achieved. Apart from all thee factors militating in favour of larger organization for animal breeding there is also pressure from commercial producers and processors. These interests, which also have grown and are growing in scale of operation, require less variation in the animals used. The numbers and quality required can be supplied only by breeders whose multiplication can offer, for example, thousands of gilts per year of the same breeding. It is not only the needs of selection which favour the large breeder but also the economics of scale of operation, multiplication and marketing, coupled with producer requirements.

Fertility

Fertility or the number of young produced at birth, is a complex character and depends not only on the number of ova shed by the female and on the amount of sperm production by the male, but also on the number of the fertilized eggs which develop properly up to the time of birth. Experiments have been made on rabbits to determine how fertility is inherited. Two low-fertility inbred strains were crossed together; these produced different numbers of eggs, one strain averaging 6 and the other 11, but much the same number at birth (average 3 and 5 respectively). The first-generation does produced double the number of young given by the parent strains. This was because the two strains crossed were of low fertility for different reasons; one strain because of the small number of eggs shed and the other strain because, although a large number of eggs were shed and fertilized, many of the embryos atrophied *in utero* before birth. The number of eggs shed behaves as a multiple factor or blending character and is just above intermediate between the two parents.

Foetal atrophy in rabbits is a maternal character, that is, it is due to the lack of some secretion in the mother's uterus and not to the genetic composition of the embryos, for females of the foetal-atrophy strain have just as much foetal atrophy when mated to unrelated males as they do with males of their own strain.

Table 4.2. Inheritance of fertility in crosses and backcrosses between two inbred lines of rabbits (H and F); results of post mortem at the 29th day of pregnancy.

Strain or cross	*No. of egg shed*	*No. of embryos*		*Atrophic embryos per 100 normals*
		Normal	*Atrophic*	
H	11.1	4.8	4.0	83.0
F	5.8	3.2	0.5	15.8
W (H×F)	10.4	6.8	1.2	17.1
U (W×W)	9.0	5.9	1.6	27.1
S (W×F)	8.2	6.7	0.4	6.0
Z (W×H)	10.3	5.7	2.8	49.1
J (Z×H)	11.3	4.4	4.4	100.0

If the pig, foetal atrophy is frequent, but there is every reason to suppose that is inherited in the same way as in rabbits, for it appears as a maternal recessive character on inbreeding. In the sheep on the other hand there is little foetal atrophy, so the number of young born depends mainly on the number of eggs she. Breeds differ considerably in this respect.

Experiments in New Zealand have shown that it is possible to increase fertility in sheep by selection. Starting in 1948 a Romney flock was divided into three groups; in one group selection was made for high fertility, in one no selection was made, and in one selection was made for low fertility. During 1948-51 the fertility percentage (lambs born per 100 ewes lambing) was 119 for the high-fertility group, 116 for the no-selection group and 100 for the low-fertility group. During 1956-9 the average fertility percentages were 137, 118 and 119 respectively and for 1967 they had advanced to 152, 119 and 108. The slow progress in the early years may have been due to absence of lifetime records of ewes from which to select rams. The rams used in succession on the flock would have far greater influence than the culling of ewes for low fertility. In the initial stages of selection before lifetime records have become available, mating the ewe lambs will, age and feeding conditions being equal, pick out those which have a high potential for fertility.

Crossing with a prolific breed, however, is a quicker method of increasing fertility in sheep. The Finnish Landrace breed which averages 2 lambs per litter for one-year-old ewes and 3 (or even more) at older ages, is now being tried out in several countries. As expected, when crossed with local breeds, fertility is intermediate.

Three seems to be no reason why twinning strains of cattle should not also be produced by selection. Possibly the best way of doing this would be to collect cows which had been recorded in the herdbooks as producing several sets of twins. Bulls to mate to those cows should be obtained from those cows which had produced several sets of twins in their lifetime, and by choosing bulls whose daughters have a high record of producing twins.

The heritability of twinning rate is low, so selection would be a very slow process. However, by using superovulation and ova transplant techniques progress could be quite fast and might increase the incidence of twins from 2 per cent to 20 per cent in a few years.

The time of onset and length of the breeding season in sheep are inherited characters which behave as intermediates on crossing. In Dorset Horns on the average the breeding season beings in July and lasts for 12 cycles as compared with November and 7 cycles in the Welsh, while the first cross begins to breed in early October and has 10 cycles.

The present understanding of the physiological mechanisms which determine genetic difference in the reproductive performance of sheep has led to the suggestion by Land that many aspects of reproductive activity in males and females are controlled, at least in part, by the

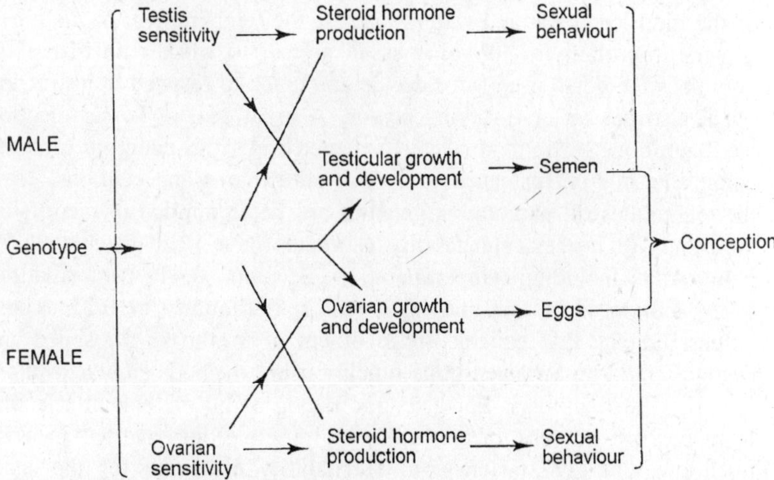

Fig. 4.1. The central role of the genadotrophic hormones in the pathway from genotype to conception in males and females.

same hormonal or metabolic variables. There is then the possibility that the reproductive or production performance of females and of a male's potential offspring can be predicted from measurements of amounts of hormones or of substances resulting from hormone action in young lambs. Similar ideas are being explored in cattle and pigs.

Horses

Horses are bred for two main purposes, speed and draught. The natural evolution of the horse is for speed and this is associated, among other things, with increase in leg length. This can be seen when fossil forms are compared on similar cranium size (ear-eye length). In the development of the individual these chances are repeated during foetal life. The proportions of the Thoroughbred form a continuation of these series and follow the normal course of evolution. Draught power requires weight and thickness of muscle and bone, which is the natural development in postnatal life, and it is by the intensification of this process that heavy breeds of horses have been developed.

It would seem that to improve the horse for speed the amount of growth early in life must somehow or other be increased, while to improve the horse for draught the development of the body after birth must be greatly increased, possibly by rearing on a high plane of nutrition such as in done in the improvement of meat animals.

In addition to the skeletal structure and the conformation, especially of the hind leg, back and rump muscles, the temperament of the horse is very important for its value as an animal to work with man. Not only does the horse need to be decide and quick to respond to instruction but it also has to have staying power. A great deal of horse selection has been done on individual performance and from pedigree records, using ancestor performance to choose elite mares and stallions. Now the techniques of quantitative genetics are being applied to records on thousands of horses. Heritability estimates have been calculated for many traits including temperament, 0.23; gaits, 0.41; conformation, 0.23; soundness of feet and legs, with a heritability of 0.35. These values indicate that genetic improvement of the horse for speed and draught could be achieved quite quickly using methods similar to those for other farm animals. For gaits and racing ability individual selection is appropriate whereas for temperament, muscling, legs and feet progeny testing would give faster gain. Heritability estimates for the same character can vary quite markedly, depending on the population on which they are calculated and the method of calculation. Wherever possible, heritability should be measured on the population being selected.

PIGS

Pigs have been bred for three main purposes—lard, pork and bacon. Lard is now of much less importance, and all three products are being obtained form the same type of pig slaughtered at different weights. For pork production, some parts of the carcase are of more value than others, so that attempts have been made to increase the proportions of the more valuable parts. As the pig grows its proportions change; during the early foetal stages the head and neck are proportionally large and the loin small but after birth, in our improved breeds, the proportions of the loin rapidly increase. When the unimproved pig, the wild boar, grows it does not change its proportions to anything like the same extent and remains, like the embryo, relatively heavy in the head and shoulders. Improvement has apparently come by selecting for increased loin development in the adult and the pushing back of this into an earlier stage of development as occurs in natural evolution. That is, such differences tend to be inherited not at a corresponding age but at an earlier age, just as the embryonic forms tend to recapitulate the evolutionary history of the breed. Thus types of pig, such as the Berkshire and the Middle White, go through these changes in proportions more quickly, and are ready for slaughter earlier, than other types, such as the Large White. That is, the character we are breeding for in the early slaughter type is a rapid change in body proportions which makes them suitable for killing at low weights. As previously pointed out, rapid change in body proportions is only possible on high nutrition and so selection is best made under conditions of good nutrition.

With this rapid change in body proportions has come an increase in those tissues, such as fat, which normally develop late in life. This is an advantage when lard is the main objective, but since the sale for this has decreased, the Poland China breed in the U.S.A. has been turned into a breed with more lean and less fat by increasing its size, and so delaying age to slaughter, as well as by changing the showyard type.

Present market requirement are for much leaner carcases than in the past. There are some differences between breeds in carcase lean content, with the Hampshire and Pietrain having good reputations for this trait. Attempts to increase the proportion of lean and reduce the proportion of fat in pork and bacon pigs by selection and by feeding and management, have sometimes increased the incidence of other problems of meat quality. In particular, when pigs have been selected for blockiness in an attempt to increase muscle to bone ratios, there has been a marked increase in pale, soft, exudative (PSE) pork and also dark firm dry (DFD) pork. These defects are probably of different genetic and environmental origins. There appears to be little relationship within British breeds between shape and lean content or proportion of high priced joints. Selection for leanness has been done by reducing fatness with less emphasis on conformation. PSE or watery pork is meat in which the red colour disappears and the muscle has poor water holding capacity. The meat is undesirable because of the weight loss and because it less suitable for curing. PSE pork is more common in pigs which are subject to stress such as caused by transport and herding just prior to slaughter. After slaughter such pigs have a rapid depletion of muscle glycogen and a low muscle pH which affects the water holding capacity. PSE condition in pigs has been shown to be closely associated with halothane-induced 'a malignant hyperthermia' syndrome. Pigs can be tested early in life by exposure to halothane gas. Those which respond can be discarded, so saving expensive test facilities. Halothane sensitivity has been shown to be due to a single gene effect.

Boars tend to grow faster, have a better feed conversion and be learner than castrates and gilts. There has therefore been much interest in leaving boars entire for pork and bacon production. However, meat processors are experiencing curing problems and excessive leanness with boars, also meat from a small proportion of boars contains an odour which can be detected, and is disliked by consumers. Research is being done to try to avoid the problem of boar odour.

In order to encourage the right system of feeding of feeding and management so that selection of pigs for commercial characters can be efficiently carried out, pig recording has been undertaken. The important records to keep are the number of pigs born and weaned to indicate the fertility and mothering quantities of the sows. In addition, the weight of the young pigs at 3 weeks old should be recorded to measure the milking qualities of the sows, for up to this time they are almost entirely dependent on the mother's milk. Weights of the young pigs can also be taken at 8 weeks of age, to measure not only the milk supply of the sow, but also the efficiency of the weaning and early rearing system adopted, because this is the critical stage in the life of the pig for obtaining length of side and efficiency of field conversion. The age at which the pig reaches slaughter weight for pork or bacon, the feed consumed and the carcase quality are also important characters to be recorded.

Table 4.3. Heritabilities of important characters in two breeds of pigs.

	Probable values	
Trait	*Large white*	*Landrace*
Growth rate (gain per day)	0.41	0.41
Feed conversion (feed/carcase gain)	0.58	0.48
Dressing out (%)	0.40	0.26
Loin length (mm)	0.46	0.39
Average backfat (mm)	0.66	0.74
Eyc musclc area	0.35	0.49

The chief means of improvement for growth and carcase characters is by progeny and performance tests, which in the past have been mainly carried out in testing stations but are now increasingly being done on breeders' own farms. Performance testing of boars has the advantage that large numbers of boars can be tested and unsuitable ones eliminated before they produce offspring. The characters that can be accurately tested in the live pig are growth rate, feed conversion, and depth of back fat (by either the probe or ultrasonic—echo-sounding—method). The latter measures the depth by the time taken for the echo to come back from the junction of fat and lean. An accurate assessment of carcase quality, particularly carcase lean, requires that a proportion of pigs be slaughtered and dissected, but this is not longer essential.

Reproductive characters such as litter size generally have low heritabilities and are very difficult to improve by within herd selection. Most of the gains in reproduction in recent years have therefore been obtained by crossbreeding and by using hybrid sows for commercial pig production. There may also be some advantages, such as enhanced libido, form using hybrid boars; but if the types included in crossbreeding are very different for growth and carcase characters the offspring from matings of hybrid sows and hybrid boars may be very variable for carcase quality.

In the U.K. in 1971 the Meat and Livestock Commission (MLC) re organized their Pig Improvements Scheme which had been operating since 1966. The revised scheme has four categories of participant, though they tend to overlap: (1) the nucleus herd; (2) the reserve nucleus herd; (3) the breeding company; and (4) the nucleus multiplier herd. The most efficient way to use this testing capacity of the MLC central stations is to make them available to a few herds at the summit of the breeding pyramid. These herds are officially designated 'nucleus'; they were chosen by an independent panel of breeders and scientists according to breeding records and management standards. They are encouraged to progeny test all their boars annually, to breed only from boars from nucleus herds, and to maintain a short generation interval. Gilt performance is tested on the farm. Reserve nucleus herds are those aspiring to become nucleus herds. After panel approval reserve nucleus herds test their pigs at MLC stations for one year at least. On the basis of the results the panel decide whether the reserve herd can be upgraded to nucleus category.

There are an increasing number of breeding companies which carry out gilt and boar testing on their own farms, but also have access for boar testing to the MLC test stations, to an extent determined by the independent panel. These companies may sell purebred and hybrid boars and gilts and may make use of breeding stock from the nucleus herds. The companies using the MLC stations also take part in the MLC Commercial Pig Evaluation Test, to compare the performance of commercial breeding stock and slaughter pigs sold by the companies.

The nucleus multiplier herds buy gilts and tested boars from the nucleus herds and multiply these for sale of purebred or crossbred stock to commercial herds. Some selection of gilts may be made in nucleus multiplier herds provided the herd users the MLC on-farm ultrasonic testing service for fat measurement. All types of herds and companies using MLC facilities must be members of the Government Pig Health Scheme.

The MLC boar performance test, or combined test as it is known, measures a young boar's potential to sire above average progeny. From any one litter of a nucleus or company herd, a test group consists of two boars on performance test and a castrate and a gilt for slaughter. During 1977-78 about 3000 boars were tested under standard feeding and management conditions in this way. The breeding value of the boars is assessed from their own performance and that of their littermates. The pigs enter the testing station when their individual weights are between 18 and 25 kg and the test starts when each boar weight 27 kg and the sibs total 54 kg. The test is completed when each boar weighs 91 kg and the sibs' total weight is 165 kg, at which time the sibs are slaughtered. Detailed carcase measurements are taken

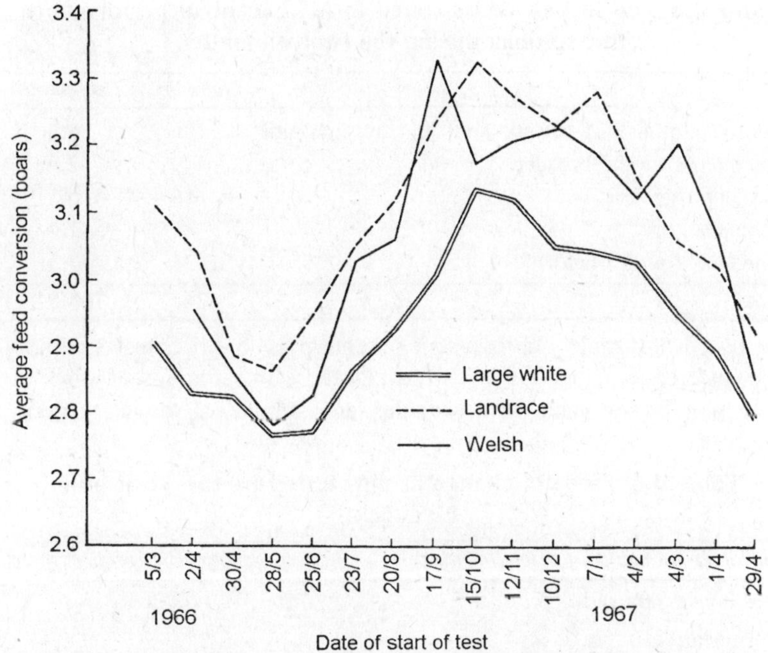

Fig. 4.2. Seasonal variation in average feed conversion by boars.

and feed consumption, live weight gain and ultrasonically measured fat depths are recorded on each boar. This information is combined with feed consumption and growth records from the sibs, plus their carcases measurements, and expressed in a selection index as a points score for each boar. In order to allow for environmental differences between different stations and at a different times of the year the two scores are presented as contemporary comparisons i.e.. they are compared with the average of other boars tested at the same station at the same time. The average score is always maintained at 100 points, although the actual performance of boars in the testing stations is improving year by year. Boars scoring below 90 points are slaughtered and boars over 90 point are offered back to the breeder. Breeders are advised to use boars with the highest scores to make the most genetic progress. Boars scoring more than 150 points are usually retained in the nucleus herd or go to an AI stud for widespread use.

The genetic progress made by the pig improvement scheme and the difference in performance between scheme pigs and those from ordinary commercial herds is mentioned regularly by MLC. Groups of pigs from specially maintained Large White and Landrace control herds

Table 4.4 The fate of boars tested in MLC central performance test stations during the twelve months.

	Number	*Percentage*
Returned for use in nucleus herd or company herd	1186	36.6
Slaughtered by the broader	420	12.9
Casualty after test	16	0.5
Incomplete test	88	2.7
Slaughtered-scores below	1534	47.3
Total	3244	100.0

are tested alongside improvement scheme pigs in MLC test stations. The difference in performance between these two sources of stock is becoming larger each year provides an estimate of annual genetic progress.

Table 4.5. Genetic change in pigs tested by the Meat and Livestock.

Character included in selection index	*Rate of genetic change per year*
Feed conversion ratio	–0.0269
Daily gain (g)	+4.91
Eye muscle area (cm^2)	+0.266
Killing out%	+0.109
Trimming%	+0.082
% lean in side	+0.683
Other characters	
Daily feed intake (g)	–7.98
'C' fat depth (mm)	–0.562
'K' fat depth (mm)	–0.692

The MLC Commercial Pig Evolution Test checks the performance of gilts and boars sold by breeding companies. Thirty hybrid gilts and seven boars are purchased on a random basis from each of nine companies and housed under commercial conditions at one test far. The test is based on the results of two litters per female; approximately 200 of the progeny of each company are fed to three different weights on two feed treatments—restricted and ad libitum. Three slaughter weights selected are 61 kg, 91 kg and 118 kg. The reproductive performance is fully recorded to provide information on number of piglets born and reared, piglet mortality and weaning weights. Feed conversion ration, daily liveweight gain and normal carcase classification measurements are recorded for the slaughter pigs. A proportion of pigs at all weights is fully dissected. Company pigs are compared with each other, with either purebred pigs or commercial crossbred gilts, and with pigs from the control herds.

In addition to these testing and selection programmes, MLC have made available since 1971 a pig carcase coalification scheme. Now some 78 percent of all pigs slaughtered (excluding sows and mature boars) are being classified. The main purpose of the information is to allocate carcases to appropriate markets and for buying purposes, but it can also be sent to the pig producer. In this way the producer can choose the type of pig and the method of feeding and management. The classification scheme is based on five factors:

1. *Cold carcase weight*;
2. *Backfat thickness*;
3. *Visual assessment* applied to certain carcases—scraggy, deformed, blemished, pigmented, coarse skinned, soft fat, pale muscle, partially condemned—these are classed as Z;

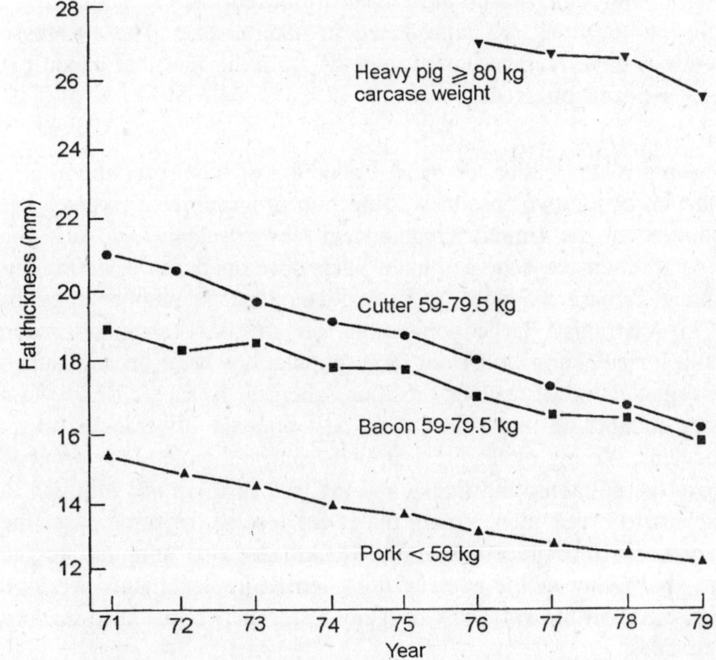

Fig. 4.3. Trends in the thickness of fat over the eye muscle in different market types of pig.

4. *Length*;
5. *Conformation*—carcases with poor conformation (particularly of the leg but not poor enough to be scraggy) are classified as C.

Measurements of thickness of subcutaneous fat over the eye muscle, at the level of the last rib, are made with an optical probe (intrascope) either 6½ cm, or both 4½ and 8 cm, from the dorsal midline (the former usually for bacon, the latter for other types of carcase).

The effect of the classification scheme on the quality of pigs being offered for slaughter has improved markedly in the eight years since it was introduced, even though carcase weights have remained almost constant.

Competition carcase tests also to some extent serve a similar purpose and were very effective in England, New Zealand and Australia in stimulating the improvement of bacon and pork pigs. In such competitions points are given so that competitors can see why their carcases do not win and so can take steps to improve them. In order to standardize inspection judging at different shows and by different judges, photographic scales have been produced. In the actual scale used the photographs are reproduced in natural size. These carcase competitions have received great impetus from the fact that bacon pig carcases are sold on grade.

Sheep

Sheep are kept either for meat production or wool production or a combination of the two products. Selection programmes for sheep has been limited in the United Kingdom; in New Zealand and Australia more comprehensive schemes have been developed for selecting for growth and carcase character, wool characters and for number of lambs born. In Australasia large populations on any one farm have been available for selection, but even large populations have been obtained by the organization of nucleus breeding schemes. In such cases several breeders collaborate and select their best animals for transfer to an elite nucleus. Young males are supplied from the nucleus for progeny testing in the collaborating flocks and the best of them are returned to the nucleus to breed more young males for testing. In some cases the best females from the collaborator flocks are also supplied to the nucleus, but many of the nucleus flock female replacements are bred in the flock form the very best progeny tested males mated to nucleus flock females.

Sheep recording is not easy to organize because of the extensive grazing conditions and limited handling which most sheep experience.

However, in 1968 MLC in the U.K. started a pilot sheep-recording scheme with the aims of discovering the problems of collecting and interpreting flock records, of establishing a series of recorded flocks throughout the country which would serve as a basis for developing local study groups, and of accumulating information for the design of possible improvement programmes. The recording scheme involves both commercial flock records and pedigree records. Several hundred flocks have participated and valuable information on comparative breed and crossbred performance, albeit under different circumstances of feeding and management, has been obtained.

The main object in breeding for improved lamb production, apart from improved lambing percentage and ewe milk yield, is to increase the proportions of the later-maturing parts of the body (e.g. loin) and the lean content of the carcase. The wild Mouflon undergoes changes in body proportions as it grows up, but in our improved breeds these have been extended in the adults, and pushed forward to an earlier stage of development, so that the body proportions of the adult Mouflon ewe are very similar to those of an improved Suffolk at 3 months old. This has apparently been done by selection in an environment of high nutrition which develops the proportions of the body to the fullest extent. All the improved early-maturing Down breeds of sheep, for example, have been produced under conditions where cultivated crops are grown and folded so that a uniform state of high plane nutrition is maintained. For fat-lamb production where the carcase has to be marketed at a low weight (15-17 kg), the early-developing parts of the body must be reduced so that more of the nutrition available goes to the later-developing parts; this, for example, means a reduction in cannon bone length and body size. Whilst it was thought that selection for early growth rate and carcase quality would have to be by progeny testing, recent research indicates that performance testing of ram lambs of Down breeds can be used to improve growth rate and fed conversion.

In order to enable the breeder to find out in what particular respect his animals are meeting, or not meeting, the requirements of the market, MLC have developed a sheep carcase chylification scheme. It is based on the four factors weight, category (lamb, hogget, or sheep), fatness as determined by a visual appraisal of external fat development, and conformation, into four classes by visual appraisal of shape, taking into account carcase thickness and blockiness and fullness of the legs. In assessing conformation fatness plays its part in influencing overall shape and no attempt is made to adjust specifically for fatness. Among carcases of similar weight and fatness, good conformation carcases tend to have greater lean meat thickness than those of poorer conformation.

Occasionally sheep occur which have yellow fat, a most undesirable character; like the similar condition in rabbits, this appears to be a simple recessive character.

Body weight tends to increase with increasing fleece weight. It should, therefore, be possible to increase meat production without detriment to wool production. Nevertheless, breeding for wool alone, as in the Merino, presents a simpler problem. For wool improvement, weight of fleece and fineness of wool fibre, among other things, are required. These are affected considerably by nutrition. Selection for fleece weight increases staple length and density (fibres per unit area) but it also increases skin wrinkles and fibre diameter. An increase in fibre diameter means a reduction in quality. Skin folds must be rigorously selected against because they lead to shearing difficulties and increased susceptibility to fly strike. Uniformity of fibre diameter over the body is said to be important but it is very difficult to measure and therefore to select for. In general, mass selection for fleece weight and wool quality gives more rapid improvement than progeny testing.

Dairy Cattle

In the conversion of the protein and energy in feeding stuffs into animal produce suitable for human consumption there is loss of nutrients. This conversion to milk by the cow is on the average more efficient than for most of the other animal products. There is, however, a great difference between individuals in this efficiency of conversion; in low-yielding cows a much higher proportion of the feed intake is required for maintenance. Since the main expense is feed, this is one of the chief reasons for breeding for high milk and butterfat production.

The selection objectives for dairy cows depend on the method of payment for milk. Whilst there has been a major emphasis on milk yield until recently, there is now more importance attached to yield of milk components such as fat and protein. Some countries such as Holland have even adopted a negative payment for increased milk volume to deter the production of water.

Most selection schemes are designed to improve milk characters but little has yet been done to select for improved efficiency of feed conversion, except by increasing yield. The look of the animal, particularly with regard to mammary structure and the quality of feet and legs—very important to a grazing animal–are included in type classification schemes which are used as additional criteria to milk characters for selection of cows and of bulls via their daughters.

Table 4.6. Heritabilities of the more important characters in dairy cattle.

Trait	*Probable values*
Milk yield	0.25–0.35
Fat yield	0.25–0.35
Protein yield	0.25–0.35
Fat percentage	0.45–0.55
Protein percentage	0.45–0.55
Total milking time	0.25–0.35
Mastitis resistance	0.20–0.35
Udder shape	0.10–0.20
Calving difficulty	0.00–0.25
Body weight	0.25–0.40

In the past the main method of improving milk yields was by milk recording and culling of the low yielders. This was wasteful because the culling is done after loss has been sustained through low milk production. The overhead food costs of rearing a heifer to milking age make the cost of milk production high if she has to be eliminated from the herd through low yield or disease before she has reached the age (7½ years) of maximum production.

Genetically, the bull must bear half the responsibility for the production of low-yielding heifers, so that better selection of the bulls used in dairy herds is a more effective and economical means of improving milk and buttefat yields than is culling the low-yielding cows'. In the past a large number of bulls were required each year because of the small average size of the herds and the short time bulls were kept in them. This position has changed. Herds are increasing in size and the use of artificial insemination, by which a bull can serve up to 80000 cows a year instead of about 35 by natural mating, means that very few bulls are now required and better selection of bulls can be made. Grading-up the commercial dairy cattle of the country by artificial insemination from proven bulls, is the first stage in the development of an improved national dairy herd. Selection schemes within breeds are the most important development now.

The bull is most important in breading for milk. No matter whether the cows in the herd are good or bad to start with, the genetic composition of the herd after four generations will depend mainly on the genetic value of the four bulls used in success in, and but slightly on the genetic make-up of the original cows. Since a bull has to be 6 years old or over before he can become progeny tested, the number of naturally proven bulls in this country is not enough to supply the requirements of artificial insemination centres. In fact the artificial insemination system is the best means of proving a bull quickly, for few herds are large enough to do this. Selection schemes are run by artificial insemination organizations and by group of private breeders.

The main difficulty met with in the progeny testing of bulls is the time it takes before the bull's breeding value for milk production is known; the bull is usually about 6 years old before the first lactation records of his daughters are available. While waiting for the results of their progeny tests bulls must be laid off; the Milk Marketing Board has over 600 bulls laid off at any time. In countries where the population to be mated by artificial insemination is under 500,000 cows it is not usually necessary or profitable to keep bulls until their progeny test results are available. A more appropriate system then is to use the bulls to produce a limited number of offspring to provide a progeny test, then to take semen from the bulls into deep freeze for perhaps a year. Up to 80,000 doses of semen may be taken from a bull in a year and this would be sufficient for use in a small population of cows. At the end of semen collection the bulls can be slaughtered, so saving maintenance costs for five years. Semen taken from bulls which subsequently have a poor progeny test result can be destroyed.

Feeding and management as well as genetics have a large influence on a heifer's yield. In order to overcome the difficulty of variation in environmental conditions on different farms, the Milk Marketing Board have adopted a method of '*contemporary comparison*' in which the first lactations of a bull's daughters are compared for the same years with those of daughters of other bulls in the same herd. In assessing the results, the actual yields of the daughters should also be taken into account, for a deceptively high index for a bull can be obtained if the other bulls with which he is compared are very poor ones. This is now done automatically in the calculation of the Improved Contemporary Comparison.

The contemporary comparison assesses a bull in terms of immediate practical interest—so much better or worse than the average bull. A good bull will be +250 kg or more; a bull poorer than average has a negative rating. The test replaces all other '*bull indexes*' and makes passible the direct comparison of all bulls of the same breed in the country. It can be used for a series of small herds—provided that there is at least one heifer by some other bull to compare with the daughters of the test bull. It gives the same results in herds with high or with low yields—thus achieving the aim for which it was invented. It is clear that the daughter averages are conditioned entirely by the herd environment and give no indication of the merit of the bull. The difference between daughters and contemporaries, on the other hand, is independent of herd level. The final justification for the contemporary comparison method of progeny testing bulls is the relationship between tests on fathers and sons. Progeny-tested bulls, when mated to average cows, produce sons whose contemporary comparisons can be predicted (with at least 70 per cent of the expected accuracy) from those of their fathers.

The accuracy of a progeny test increases with the number of daughters, rapidly until the number reaches 20-25, after which additional daughters increase the accuracy more slowly. With the contemporary comparison the effective number of daughters is a weighted number rather less than the actual number of daughters. For instance, 30 actual daughter give a 'weight' of about 20 effective daughters, i.e. they give as much information as would 20 daughters all milking together in one herd and compared against a large number of daughters by other bulls. The Milk Marketing Board publishes the contemporary comparison of bulls who have a minimum of 20 effective daughters.

For buttefat percentage, daughter averages are satisfactory because, unlike milk production, this does not vary so much with feeding conditions. Naturally the yields of all and not some selected daughters of a bull should be used in calculating the progeny test.

The difficulty of environmental differences between farms can also be overcome by feeding 20 heifers, from each of several bulls to be tested, on standard rations on the same farm, as is done in Denmark, where the heifers are brought to the testing station a month or so before they are due to calve. This method was adopted by the British Oil and Cake Mills at Selby. It was found, however, that the heifers varied considerably in condition owing to different systems of rearing on the various farms from which they came. Because of this they tried bringing them in as calves, so that the heifers from different bulls would all be reared under similar conditions, a system which is used in Iceland. In countries with a large herd size, progeny testing stations are a much more expensive form of testing than the use of farm records. However, in countries with small herds progeny testing stations or special nucleus recording herds may be the only effective means of bull selection.

When good 'proven' bulls are obtained, full use should be made of them for the improvement of dairy cattle, particularly by breeding further bulls for testing. These must be red out of cows with a long lifetime record of high production. Because some high-yielding cows transmit their high yields better than others, an additional safeguard is to choose a cow which has produced high-yielding daughters. If bulls are selected in this way the next generation should produce animals not only with high yields but also with a long life and a good constitution. This is supported by New Zealand results which show that the best method of selecting a young dairy bull is to take a son of a proven sire out of a cow with a long lifetime record of high production, particularly if she has already produced good milking daughters. By this means one is breeding not only for production but also for constitution and livability, both essential factors in commercial milk production.

The chief criterion used in culling cows, and in progeny testing bulls, is milk yield—usually the contemporary-day first-lactation yield. The emphasis should be on the first lactation for the following reasons:

1. The first lactation gives a reasonably good indication of lifetime yield, i.e. repeatability of yield is fairly high.
2. Heritability of first lactation yield is higher than that of second lactation, i.e. the first lactation is less influenced by environmental factors (e.g. preceding dry period) and is thus a better indictor of a cow's genetic capacity.
3. In progeny testing, only for the first lactation it is possible to obtain a group of unselected daughters of a bull.
4. The results are available much sooner than if later lactations are awaited.

With some exceptions, which must be watched, bulls selected on the basis of first lactations are still the best bulls when judged on second and third lactations.

Owing to the negative correlation between milk and fat percentage, selection for milk yield will tend to lower fat percentage. This negative correlation is less for second lactations and disappears in later ones. The trend can be kept in check by culling low-fat heifers and bulls while maintaining the main selection pressure on yield.

The colour of the milk and buttefat has become important economically since milk has been sold in bottles. The colour is due to carotin, which is formed form the pigment associated with the green colouring matter of plants. In some breeds such as the South Devon, Guernsey and Jersey the colour of the body fat and butterfat is well developed, whereas in many individuals of the other dairy and beef breeds the pigment is broken down in the liver and the fat is pale in colour.

In cattle this is probably a multiple-factor or blending character because all shades exist. In the absence of green food in the ration, all breeds produce butterfat dead-white in colour. As the amount of green food in the ration is increased so the intensity of the colour increases to a maximum, which varies with the individual and bred, beyond which no amount of additional greenstuff will increase the colour. Thus, as for many other commercial characters, it is impossible to select and breed for butterfat colour unless optimum conditions are given for its formation.

In breeding tropical cattle for milk production 'temperament' is one of the factors to be considered. Milk is 'let down' by a reflex oxytocin discharge set up by suckling or stroking the teats. In the early days of domestication, and in unimproved herds today, this reflex will not take place except in the presence of the calf. By selecting for a take place except in the presence of the calf. By selecting for a docile temperament, milk is set down without the presence of the calf. As has been shown by experiments in Jamaica and Trinidad, this character is inherited and can be transmitted through the bull.

Buffalo

In many parts of the world, but especially in Asia, the buffalo is an important animal for draught, for milk production and to a lesser extent for meat. There are about 140 million domesticated water buffaloes of two main types termed the Swamp and the River Buffalo, which will interbreed though they have different chromosome number. The former is predominantly a drought animal of the rice areas of the Far East whilst the latter is a dairy animal mainly found in India and Pakistan. There are many herds of buffalo ranging from 250 kg to 1000 kg mature weight. Milk production may vary from low yields of 1500 kg to high yields of over 500 kg in lactations extending to 400 days. Buffalo milk contains more fat and protein than cows milk. The buffalo female reaches puberty and sexual maturity later than cattle heifers of European or tropical breeds, and has a longer gestation period of between 300 and 330 days. The heritabilities of characters such as fertility, milk production and composition and growth rate in buffalo are thought to be similar to those for the same characters in cattle. Buffaloes have less variation in body colour and there has been less interest in establishing breed societies and herdbooks than for cattle. Most buffalo are kept in small herds and artificial insemination is not widespread. For these and other reasons there have been few attempts to select the buffalo for important commercial characters. It is reasonable assumption that selection methods which have been successful with cattle will be equally appropriate for buffalo. Thus improvement of fertility may be achieved by crossbreeding to benefit from hybrid vigour, and of growth rate can be based on performance testing and individual selection. Improvement of carcase quality would have to include some progeny testing. Milk yield and quality can be improved by progeny testing males on the first lactation records of their daughters. Small farm herd size lack of AI and of recording may make this difficult except in large herds especially established for the purpose, as with the dairy cattle progeny testing stations in Denmark. In far herds individual selection for milk yield has been tried but the rate of gain has been low and of the order of 0.1 per cent year. Genetic gains of 0.5 to 1.0 per cent per year can be expected in schemes in large herds using progeny testing.

Beef Cattle

Most of the beef in the world is produced form purebred and cross bred beef cattle. Beef cows are grazed under extensive, often hard and poor, range conditions and mated by mated by natural service by bulls running with the cows on range. The calves produced are usually weaned at 6 months to a year and may be raised to slaughter either on improved pasture or on silage and concentrate feeds in a feedlot. Selection has been concerned mainly with improving the growth and carcase character of the bulls used, so that their offspring will perform better on pasture or on feedlot. It is difficult to select for improved beef cows because recording the performance of cows is not easy under range conditions. What little selection has been done has concentrated on selecting those cows which produce the greatest weight of weaned calf per year. Such a selection criterion is a composite of several characters including fertility of the cow, calf survival and growth, and cow milk yield to the calf.

Choice of breed allows selection of breed of cow, which can cope with the particular range conditions, and of breed of bull, which can survive to mate cows on range and produce fast growing, good carcase, calves for slaughter. Under many circumstances the choice of cows and bulls involves at least two breeds and sometimes three or more. Many of the cows are the cross of two breeds in order to obtain the benefits of hybrid vigour for reproductive characters and calf survival. A very large breed comparison is in progress at the U.S. Department of Agriculture Clay Center, Nebraska, in which the main beef purebreeds and crossbreeds are being assessed for the important beef characters.

In Europe beef production from beef-bred cattle (purebred or crossbred) is limited mainly to the marginal land, for the overhead charges on breeding cows on good land are too high under the one-calf one-cow system of rearing. Production of a twinning breed of beef cattle would, as in the case of sheep, reduce these overhead charges, but until this is done most of our beef must be supplied from other sources.

A large amount of beef in Europe, particularly in the U.K., comes from dairy cows which are either purebred (mainly Friesian) or crossbred (beef breed sire × Friesian cow). The calves used in this form of production are a by-product of the dairy industry. Though in the U.K. these calves have been mainly steers, the majority in mainland Europe are bulls because they produce leaner carcases to suit market needs and because they grow faster and convert feed to meat more efficiently. Improved methods of rearing will do much to reduce the costs of production and the quantity and quality of beef from dairy calves. By using first crosses, however, it is possible to utilize the poorer dairy cows to breed cattle suitable for beef. Not all the cows in a diary herd are required to breed replacement heifers, and if in a herd of 100 cows 60 are inseminated by a good dairy bull the 40 worst can be inseminated by a good beef bull to supply calves for beef purposes. By such methods the dams of the replacements of the dairy herd are a selected and the culls used for beef. For such a system of corresponding, the beef breeds most often used are those like the Hereford, Charolais and Aberdeen Angus, which have dominant characters and so colour-mark their calves. The Charolais and the Simmental are particularly useful for increasing growth when crossed on the smaller dairy breeds. In buying suckler weaned calves, a premium is paid for white-faced or yellow-dum coloured calves because it is clear that they are sired by a beef bull.

In these beef production systems it is possible to improve beef characters by selecting for better beef breed sires for crossbreeding.

In addition it may be possible to select for beef as well as milk characters in dairy cows. However, the benefits of this are by no means proven. Faster growth rate in dairy cows may lead to larger cows with a higher feed maintenance but not necessarily with a proportionately higher milk yield. The improvements for beef may therefore be less than the losses in fed conversion for milk. Therefore beef improvement is best concentrated on selection of beef breed sires.

The most important characters to determine profitable production in beef cattle are growth rate, feed consumption and conversion, and carcase quality. The heritabilities of these characters are medium to high and the same principles of selection hold as in breeding for lamb and pig meat. Growth rate of beef cattle can be measured in both cows and bulls. Beef cattle are often kept in small herds and their generation interval is already long. Performance and progeny test facilities are not interchangeable. Therefore growth rate can be most rapidly improved by mass selection (or individual selection, which is the same thing). In view of the small size of herds, breeders need to buy-in bulls to avoid inbreeding. To compare their own bulls with those from other herds their growth rate must be compared under the standard conditions of a performance-testing station.

There is therefore no case for progeny testing 'breeders bulls' for growth rate. There may be a case for progeny testing them for carcase characters, but only if the progeny test can be obtained form field records. It would not justify building special progeny-testing stations or detracting from performance-testing facilities.

The heritability of weight gain is fairly high. Therefore the bulls' own performance gives a reasonably accurate estimate of his breeding value for growth. Rate of gain is correlated with efficiency of feed utilization so that, according to Pierce *et al.* (1954) for each increase of 0.1 kg again per day over the average, 23 kg digestible nutrients for each 100 kg liveweight are saved. According to Swiger *et al.* (1965) selection for 'final weight alone is 90 per cent as efficient as a selection index including weaning weight, post weaning gain, feed consumption and fatness of carcase, but feed consumption and fatness would increase'. Hence the importance of measuring feed consumption in the performance test. If carcase qualities are also important, a progeny test must be employed at present. However, research is in progress to find ways, such as ultrasonic techniques and body scanners, of measuring carcase quality in the live animal, and if successful this would largely do away with the need for progeny tests.

Performance testing of beef bulls can be carried out in three ways. The first, known as time constant testing, involves measuring the animals growth rate over a certain time period, say of 150 or 200 days, irrespective of the age and weight of the individual animals at start of test. The second method, weight constant testing, is the measurement of the time it takes for animals to grow over a specified weight range, for example from 250 to 400 kg. The third method, age constant testing, is the weight gain of animals over a specified age range such as 150 to 400 of age. For each method it is possible to measure feed intake. The second method has several advantages, particularly if the weight range forest is equivalent to the weight range for commercial beef animals. Poor performing animals can be culled at an early stage in the test if performance in early test is closely related to final result. This means that more animals can be tested in the facilities available and the generation interval may also be reduced. In the United Kingdom but performance tests are run by the Meat and Livestock Commission at 5 stations, accommodating in total about 400 bulls annually. Growth rate and feed intake of individual bulls is measured, using age constant testing for a period from about 150 to 400 days of age. The whole period of the test is considered as an equilibrating period during which the effects of different farm treatments before weaning and start of test can wear off. In the U.S.A., time constant testing is used in which bull calves are taken at weaning from their dams and, under uniform conditions of feeding, rate of gain and feed consumption is measured for 140, 196 and 240 days. At the end of test the bulls are classified according to conformation and finish. The full effect of performance testing on breed improvement can only be obtained when the best of the tested bulls are used to breed young bulls for testing in the next generation.

Tradition has favoured selection in a high nutrition environment, on the theory that this will show the extend to which more valuable parts of the carcase are capable of developing. Under range conditions where feeding is often poor after weaning, little progress is apparent from breeding, and such areas import bulls regularly to keep up the beef qualities of their stock. These bulls are produced instead farms under conditions of unlimited nutrition, nurse cows frequently being used until they are about 18 months old so that proper selection can be made of bulls which show greatest development of beef qualities. One disadvantage of this system is that the bulls which grow best under conditions of intensive feeding are not necessarily the ones whose progeny grow best under more extensive conditions. In the U.K. it is probably satisfactory to performance test bulls on a high concentrate ration because their progeny, though on pasture, can also experience a high nutritional plane. But bulls selected in this way will probably not give the progeny best adapted to dry tropical ranges.

In the United Kingdom the MLC, in addition to performance testing stations, has provided a beef recording system used both by pedigree breeders and by commercial beef producers. This system has provided comparative breed information on growth rate. Comparisons of feed conversion for breeds and crossbreeds cannot usually be obtained from farm records, so the MLC have set up two Commercial Beef Evaluation Units for this purpose and have also obtained much information on breed carcase quality.

For a beef production system growth rate is closely related to profitability. The growth rates of different breeds of bull are a good indication of the comparative weight of their offspring from suckler cows and in the U.K. the ranking of breed performance is much the same irrespective of the farm type.

The choice of beef bulls for use in artificial insemination presents different problems. At the moment they are used almost exclusively to produce commercial beef cattle—either crossbred breeding females or steers for slaughter. This means that criteria such as rate of genetic improvement are inapplicable. The maximum economic advantage will come from selecting accurately the bulls transmitting the economically important characters of growth rate, feed-utilization efficiency and carcase quality, and using them on a large scale.

The Milk Marketing Board in England and Wales has a special farm for progeny testing its beef bulls used for artificial insemination, and the Meat and Livestock Commission is using the records from its beef-recording service to progeny test other bulls used in artificial insemination.

The progeny test is easier to apply in beef than in dairy cattle, for beef qualities are visible in both sexes and at all ages, so that beef bulls can be proven at a much earlier age than dairy bulls. In progeny testing for beef, at least 20 steers from each bull are taken at weaning for beef breeds, and as calves for dairy breeds, and reared, preferably by individual feeding, under similar conditions, an appraisal is made of their carcases at slaughter. In these tests the question arises as to whether the steers should be killed at a certain degree of finish, at a certain age or at a certain weight. The first criterion is difficult to estimate; the second is easy to operate but may give some carcases which are too fat (or heavy) and some that are too lean (or light); the third has the advantage that carcase measurements can then be compared directly as in pig progeny testing, and is more comparable to commercial practice.

One of the chief difficulties in making progeny tests for beef is in evaluating the carcase qualities. The MLC have introduced a beef carcase classification scheme. The carcases are described by the following characteristics:

1. *Weight*—to include or exclude kidney, knob and channel fat
2. *Sex* — steer, heifer, cow or bull
3. *Fatness*—based on one of five fat classes according to the level of fat cover, with 1 indicating the leanest and 5 the fattest class. Class 3 is subdivided into 3L and 3H, with low and higher fat content.
4. *Conformation*—based on one of five classes with 5 indicating very good and 1 indicating poor conformation. About 1 percent of carcases are very poor and classed as Z. The class is determined by a visual appraisal of shape, taking into account carcase thickness and blockiness and fullness of the round. Fatness is not taken into account.

Classification is carried out by experienced staff to a national standard. About 21 per cent of carcases in 1979 were classified as average, 3L fatness 3 conformation. The market in the U.K. is tending to require a carcase with a classification of 2 fatness 4 conformation, with the European market requiring even leaner carcases and the U.S. market requiring fatter ones.

Poultry

In breeding for egg production the chief means of improvement is the progeny test. This is particularly so in the case of cocks in which production cannot be measured directly. For example, it has been found better to breed from a hen which herself only produces say 150 eggs. Usually the progeny test is modified into a sib test; that is, instead of waiting for the results of a progeny test a son of a progeny-tested code is used, i.e. the brother (sib) of high-producing hens. Hens are selected according to their own yield and that of their sisters. Breeding from progeny-tested cocks and hens also ensures selection for constitution and livability, qualities which have been much neglected in the poultry industry in the past. Since such methods are costly and laborious, they are usually confined to large-scale breeders who supply breeding stock to those who are producing eggs for hatcheries, which in turn distribute day-old chicks to commercial producers.

Naturally many different qualities go to build up high egg production, a constitution suited to the environment not being the least important.

Egg production has increased under selection chiefly by reduction in the age at first egg (earlier sexual maturity) but also by increase in intensity of lay (reduction in broodiness and in laying pauses). Unfortunately, as egg yield increases egg size tends to decline, owing to the negative genetic correlation between these two traits. Egg weight must therefor be considered in selection as well as egg number. To increase efficiency of feed use, body weight must be held constant or reduced. Shell thickness is also important and, to a less extent, internal egg quality—firmness of white and absence of blood and meat spot.

Yolk colour, like butterfat colour previously mentioned, is an inherited character, and can be bred for in the same way. In Europe dark yolks are preferred, in America light ones. Shell colour is also inherited and is probably controlled by several pairs of genes, some of them acting cumulatively to produce darker shades. In Britain, brown shells are preferred; in most of the U.S.A. and the Mediterranean area, white ones.

For commercial egg production crosses are now widely used, as the hybrid vigour of the first cross usually gives a high uniform level of egg production. For obtaining this hybrid vigour, however, much depends on crossing two or more strains which 'nick' well, that is, which contain characters complementary to one another. Such strains can be built up by progeny testing the cocks of one breed on the hens of the other breed, and then breeding such progeny-tested cocks back to hens of their own breed to produce a strain which will give good results when crossed with the other breed. This is known as recurrent selection.

In recent years the broiler industry has increased greatly. For this a bird of 1 to 2 kg at 7 to 9 weeks old is produced by feeding on a ration with a high energy content. This has entailed selection for rapidly-growing and plump-breasted strains. Broilers must also have white plumage and rapid feathering to avoid the dark marks of unerupted feathers under the skin. White skin and legs are preferred in Britain, yellow skin and legs in America. White legs are dominant to yellowlegs; this is a simple segregating character and can easily be manipulated.

For both egg and broiler production, crossing is the usual breeding system. This may be a simple 2-way cross (A × B) but more usually it is necessary to employ a 3-way cross (A × BC) or a 4-way cross (AB × CD) to ensure that the dams (or both parents) are crossbreds and therefore the maximum benefit from hybrid vigour is gained in the multiplication of stocks for commercial sale.

INBREEDING

The mating together of close relatives, or inbreeding, not only makes more homozygous the germ-plasm and qualities of those animals which are inbred, but it also brings to light any recessive mutations which the strain of animals has in its germ-plasm.

The rapidity of the degree to which the germ-plasm is made homozygous and the uniformity of the animals obtained, depends on the closeness of the inbreeding; this comes in the following order—full brother to full sister or parent to offspring; half-brother to half-sister or grandparent to grand-child; nephew to aunt or niece to uncle; first cousins. The essential in inbreeding is an ancestor common to both parents. The farther back in the pedigree the common ancestor lies, the less intense is inbreeding.

Linebreeding, although often used to mean 'mild inbreeding' is, correctly, the form of inbreeding based on a sing common ancestor, for example a sire whose sons, grandson and great-grandson are used in succeeding generations. It may be successful, not because it is a form of inbreeding, but because of the exceptional merit of the animal on which the linebreeding is based. Its advantages are that a high degree of uniformity of type and production is attained in the herd. One form of linebreeding which has been successfully used with cattle is that of using home-bred rather than purchased bulls the home-bred bulls being taken in turn form different cows which are known to have bred well.

When after a time it is observed that the breeding has become too close, the first sings of this usually being a drop in milk yield and slow growth of the young animals, the best way to introduce new blood without disturbing types type is to obtain a bull with 50 percent outside blood. That is, to go to a good herd to which a good bull has been sold and buy a young bull sired by him out of an old high-producing cow which has already produced good milking daughters. To obtain new blood for beef herds which have become too inbred, and to prevent type being broken, the best way is to buy some good heifers and mater them with the herd bull. After noting how their offspring blend with the herd-type, a young herd bull can be bred from the heifers which breed nearest to the desired type.

By inbreeding, all recessive mutations lying hidden within the strain are brought to light. What these defects are will vary with each strain of animal inbred. For example, in two of four different strains of rabbits each inbred over some 20 generations few, if any, defective characters were seen, while in the other two strains a number of defective recessive mutations such as hypospadias, spina bifida, furlessness and foetal atrophy appeared, but could be weeded out by selective breeding. These defects appear more frequently in inbreeding than in random mating because under inbreeding conditions the same allele is more likely to be present in both parents; defects are more likely to be recessive than dominant, so the same mutation has to be present in both parents before it can show itself.

Because of the many recessive genes with small negative effects on vigour, inbreeding invariably leads, in the long run, to inbreeding depression or degeneration. Apart from specific defective mutations, the first signs of loss of commercial characters due to inbreeding appear in poor mothering qualities of the dam, loss of fertility, reduced

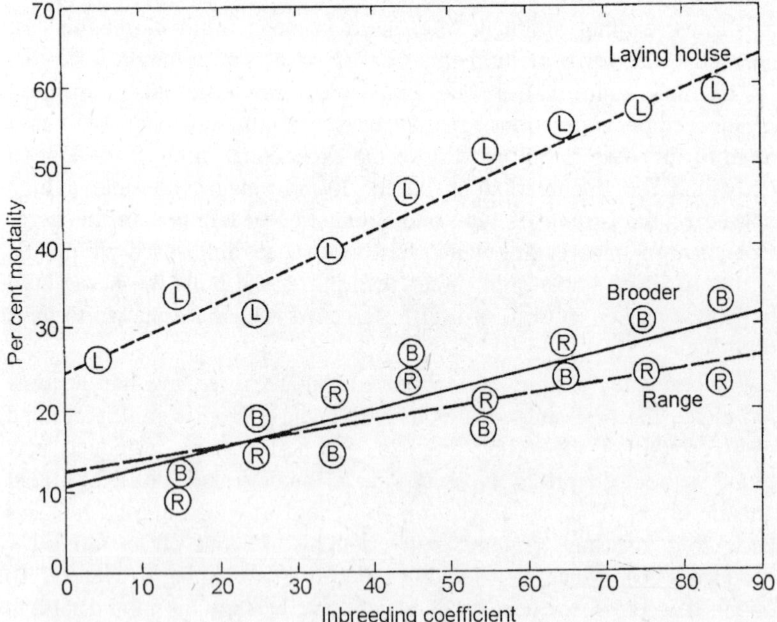

Fig. 4.4. Effects of inbreeding on viability of chickens.

milk production and slow growth of the young. Characters of less importance for survival, for example butterfat percentage, egg weight, and carcase characters, are less affected by inbreeding. King (1967), for example, found that while outbred Large White gilts produced on the average 10.2 young and weaned 8.3 each of 13.3 kg weaning weights, litters from 44 per cent inbred gilts averaged only 7.6 at birth and 5.6 weaned, with a weaning weight of 10.8 kg. For this reason, it is advisable, when exploiting hybrid vigour by crossing inbred lines, to use as female a cross between two inbred lines while using an inbred male. A male inbred for good qualities will breed better than he looks, whereas an outbred male will not breed as well as his appearance suggests. In the performance testing of males this has to be taken into account.

The first effect in inbreeding is to sieve out all the recessive genes that the animals contain so that these characters make their appearance usually in the first to third generation of inbreeding. Thus the first result of inbreeding is usually to cause increased variation in the offspring. If, however, proper selection of like types is made at this stage and inbreeding with the selected animals is continued, true breeding types will be obtained. For example, the top line the range of variability normally found in lambs' tails in a Romney flock, ranging form those in which the good spreads about half-way down the tail to those in which the hair extends to seven-eighths up to the length of the tail. On inbreeding the extent of the variability increases due to the segregation of the recessive genes.

Some of these recessive genes give rise to tails in which the good wool extends almost to the tip and other recessive genes give rise to tails which are hairy right up to the top of the tail. If selection is now made and a ram and ewes with good wool tails are mated together they will breed true for this character and the variability in the tails will be reduced. The same thing will happen if the lambs with hairy tails are bred together. This experiment demonstrates that inbreeding decreases the variation within inbred lines while increasing the variation between them.

The chances of obtaining the characters one requires on inbreeding are much increased if one inbreeds to progeny-tested sires or dams, that is, those which are known to have a large number of the desired genes. This was, in fact, the method used by the pioneer breeders, as the following pedigree of the noted Shorthorn bull Comet bred by Collings shows:

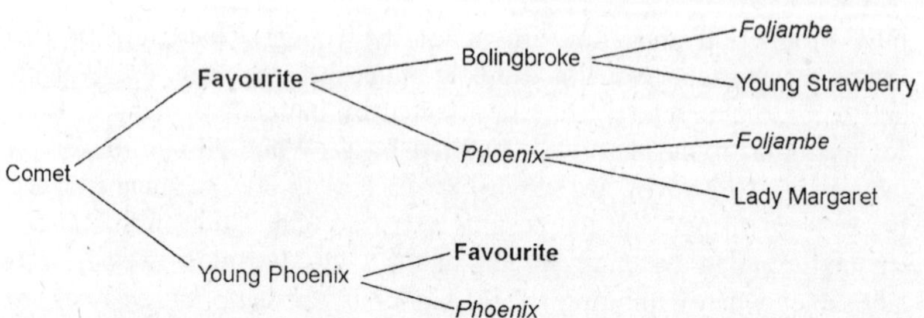

However, the inbreeding in the early history of the Shorthorn breed apparently also led to low fertility.

Studbooks, Herdbooks and Flockbooks

When beginning directive breeding for any particular object it is necessary first of all to find and then to concentrate the germ-plasm which contains the genes necessary for the development of the characters required. Studbooks, herdbooks and flockbooks have been established to segregate selected animals and breed them together, so ensuring that their germ-plasm is not diluted with the germ-plasm of unregistered stock. This concentration of the blood of strains showing the most desirable qualities involves restriction in the number of parents and hence inevitably leads to some inbreeding. Measurements of the coefficients of inbreeding show that with the passing of time the animals recorded in a studbook become more and more inbred. Many of our herdbooks have now grown so large, however, that progress in concentrating the best germ-plasm is slow, and therefore some herdbook

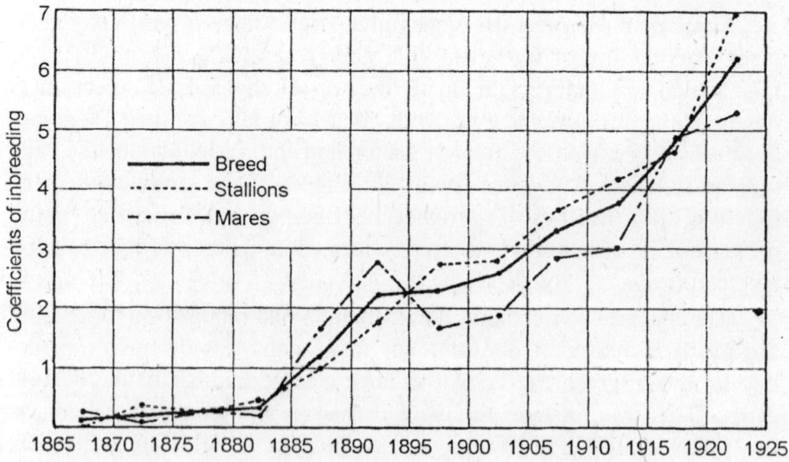

Fig. 4.5. Average percentage of inbreeding of horses.

authorities are forming an '*inner circle*' of animals with the best records—'*advanced registers*' within the herdbook—and it is from these animals that most of the sires used in the breed come.

Studies made on herdbooks show that in many breeds there is a stratification of herds. At the top are those of constructive breeders who are actively improving their cattle; they sell bulls to other pedigree breeders who multiply their stock and sell bulls to commercial producers. This is very evident in a breed such as the Friesian, where bulls have been imported. Recently, however, by the use of artificial insemination, it has been possible to shortcut this process by using bulls from constructive breeders direct on commercial cattle.

In interpreting the value of a pedigree from a herdbook, too much weight should not be placed on the performance of animals far back in the pedigree. The sire and dam each contribute half the germ-plasm of the animal, the grandparents one-quarter each the great-grandparents one-eighth each and so on back in each successive generation. Figure also illustrates how it is that, if the value of the sire and dam is known, more distant ancestors cannot give further information because their contribution to the individual's germ-plasm is included in that of the parents.

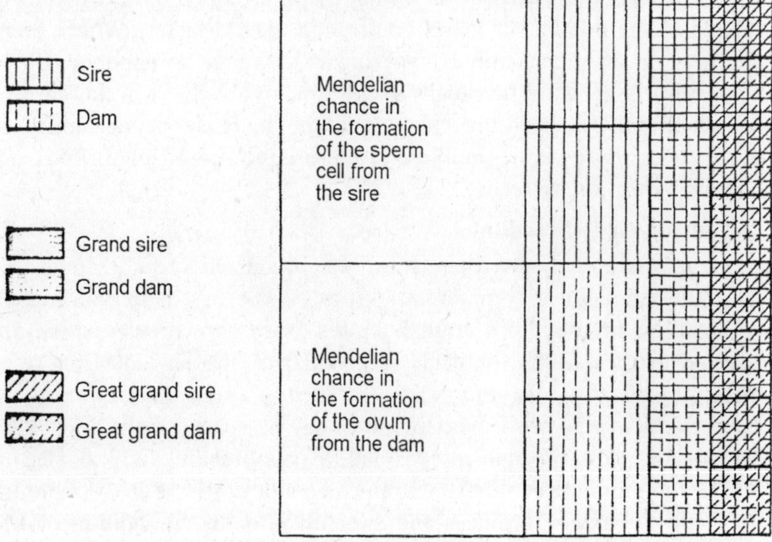

Fig. 4.6. Relative part played by the different ancestors in the genetic make-up of an animal as calculated from the Mendelian theory when random breeding is practised.

CROSSBREEDING

Cross breeding does exactly the opposite of inbreeding. In the first cross the dominant genes of the two breeds crossed mask the recessive genes. The first cross animal usually exhibits hybrid vigour because the recessive characters tend to be the less desirable ones. When, however, such first crosses are mated together, increased variability in appearance results because the recessive characters segregate again, so that animals may appear with the characters of both parent breeds. For example, in crosses between Aberdeen-Angus and Hereford cattle, the black face of the Aberdeen-Angus and the horns of the Hereford behave in inheritance as do many of the bad characters of the animal and disappear in the first cross, which gives an animal with all the dominants of both breeds and so a superior animal for beef purposes. When, however, these first crosses are bred are produced. This can also be illustrated by some experiments made by crossing dogs of different type. For example, if the Boston terrier be taken as representing dairy type of animal and the Dachsund be taken as representing a beef-type animal, then the result of the first cross is a super animal. But if such crosses are interbred, segregation of types occurs in the second generation.

However, the increase in variability on crossbreeding is inversely related to the number of genes controlling the character. Where there are few, as in the example involving colour and horns, increase in variability is great. When many genes are involved, as in the case of the quantitative, economic characters, the increase in variability of the F_2 over the F_1 is negligible and there is no reason to shrink from breeding from crossbreeds.

Organized Crossbreeding

There are to main reasons for the organized crossbreeding of domestic animals for commercial purposes. The first is to obtain good commercial returns from animals culled from pure breeds which are adapted to special environments (e.g. hills) or special industries (e.g. milk production). In the animal industry there is frequently a '*stratification of types*', both in time and in space, from poor low-priced land to good high-priced land. Cross-breeding is practised to bridge the gap between these extremes economically. For example, in poor hilly country hardiness and suitability to their condition of life are the main considerations for the economic success of sheep; here is the place of the Blackface breed in Scotland. The cull ewes drafted from the hill flocks of this breed are taken to slightly better land where they are mated with rams of the crossing breeds such as the Border Leicester which are of larger size and are commonly regarded as being more fertile and having a higher milk yield. The males of this cross, the Greyface, are reared for slaughter, and the females are sent to the good pasture land in the north of England, where their progeny by the rams of the specialized meat breeds such as the Suffolk and Hampshire Down are sold as fat lambs.

A similar stratification holds in Australia. The cull Merino ewes (toothless grannies) from the pastoral areas, plus some cull Merino '2-tooths', are taken to the wheat belt and crossed with Border Leicester rams, their female progeny going to the subterranean-clover or irrigated areas to be mated with Dorset Horn or Polled Dorset rams for the production of fat lamb. The qualities of hardiness, good fertility and good milk supply are brought in from the ewe, while good mutton qualities are brought in from the ram. Likewise in New Zealand the cull Romney ewes from the hills are mated to Southdown rams to produce lambs which are sold from the low-country pastures as fat lamb.

The second reason for crossbreeding is to exploit hybrid vigour by crossing two lines, strains or breed and thus obtain a strong, vigorous, high producing animal for commercial production in species, such as pigs and poultry, in which the breeding stock can easily be replaced. Thus in breeding fowls first crosses are made between two different breeds or strains. These are mated to a third breed or strain or to another first cross to produce vigorous second-cross birds for egg or meat production. A refinement of this crossbreeding for egg production is to inbreed the parent strains before crossing, as has been successfully done with maize. Many inbred lines are produced and many crosses made between them in pairs. Only the best crosses are exploited commercially, i.e. those lines which 'nick' best on crossing are retained.

While the first signs of lack of vigour on inbreeding are seen in the mothering qualities of the am, so in reverse the most striking effects of crossbreeding are the increase in the fertility and milk yield of the dam and in the rate of growth of the young. Crossbreeding for meat purposes is based partly on the fact that good growth rate and early maturity depend on a good milk supply. This is particularly so with beef cattle, where many of the pedigree bulls are reared on nurse cows and so are not selected for quick growth based on milk supply from their own dam. Hence in Britain commercial beef herds usually consist of first-cross cows mated back to a bull of one or other of the parent breeds or to one of a third breed. Experiments in U.S.A. have shown that when Hereford cows were mated with

Shorthorn bulls and their offspring put to Aberdeen-Angus bulls the calves weighed 212 kg at weaning as compared with an average of 176 kg for the pure breeds, and on similar feeds gave a final weight of 469 kg as compared with 414 kg for the pure breeds. Similar results have been found in a large comparison involving temperate and tropical cattle and large breeds such as the Charolais and China, conducted at the Roman L. Hruska U.S. Meat Animal Research Center, Nebraska.

When British beef breeds are crossed the average of the two reciprocal crosses is better than the average of the two parent breeds by about 5 per cent for growth and viability and about 8 per cent for cow fertility. When British breeds are crossed with Zebus the amount of hybrid vigour is two or three times as great.

The same thing applies to pig breeding. If the full advantage is to be made of hybrid vigour, crossbred females should be used as breeders. Table 4.7 shows the percentage advantages obtained form the first-cross litters and from litters of the first-cross sows by a boar of a third breed over those of the pure breeds concerned for different characters. It is evident that in birth weight per litter, number of pigs born and weaned, and weight at weaning, there is great advantage in using the first-cross sow. In many parts of the world pig production for pork and bacon is based on crosses of two, three or four strains or breeds. As with poultry the identity of breeds has been lost in most of the crossbreeds used. Breeds of pigs such as Middle White, Tamworth, Berkshire and Welsh have declined to minor importance and most crossbreeds are based on Large White, Landrace, with introductions of Hampshire, Duroc and the Belgian Pietrain.

Table 4.7. Percentage advantages of pigs in first-cross litters over purebreds and compared with those bred from first-cross sows mated with a boar of another breed.

	First cross from purebred sow	*Second cross from first-cross sow*
Birth weight per live pig	1.96	0.39
Birth weight per litter of live pigs	13.39	26.65
Number of live pigs per litter	11.22	20.19
Total number of pigs per litter	4.04	8.62
Number of pigs weaned per litter	5.87	36.22
Litter weight at weaning	24.84	60.76
Saving in feed	2.99	3.85
Saving in time to reach 100 kg	8.67	8.63

In general, to obtain the full benefits from hybrid vigour it is essential to exploit the increased fertility and mothering ability of the crossbred females. This may be done by mating them to a third breed and slaughtering all the offspring for meat as described above, or by using a criss-crossing system, i.e. using sires of the two breeds in alternate generations. This retains hybrid vigour (or at least two-thirds of it) but it simpler in that only one kind of breeding female is kept instead of two—one pure and one crossbred.

Replacement crossing (or grading up) and the formation of new breeds also involve breeding from crossbred females, but after the first cross, do not efficiently exploit hybrid vigour.

Grading Up

Replacement crossing enables us to improve low-producing stock rapidly by mating them, and their progeny in several successive generations, with purebred males of a highly productive strain. This process is known as *grading up*. In the course of about four generations bred in this way one can obtain animals which will be indistinguishable in appearance and performance and will breed almost as well as the purebred animals to which they were graded. This is especially so if the males used for grading purposes come in each generation from the same strain, or the grade females are inbred in successive generations

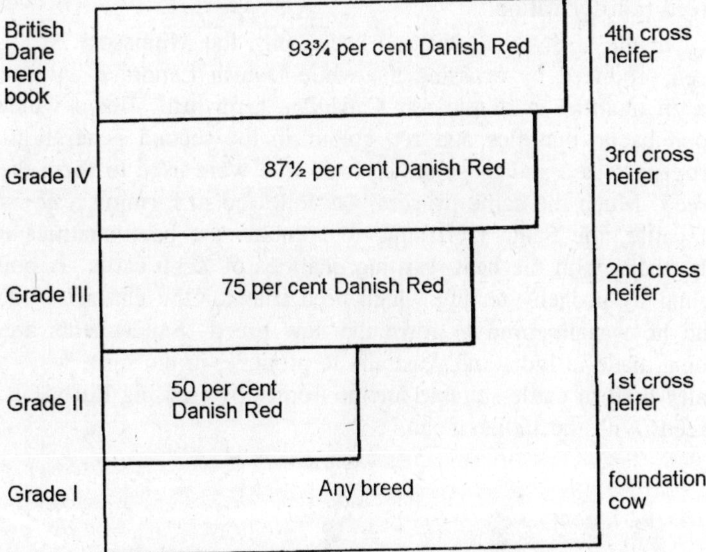

Fig. 4.7. Diagram showing how the grading-up scheme of the Red Poll Cattle.

to the same purebred male. This method is now being used to replace one breed by another or to introduce the polled character into horned breeds of cattle.

Formation of New Breeds

With plants the production of new varieties has been brought about by crossing two strains, each with some desirable character which it was desired to combine. The same system is used to form new breeds of animals. Where the breeds crossed do not differ materially in the unit factor characters or fancy points, it is easy to establish new breeds which have the mean values of their commercial characters lying at any point between those of the two parents crossed, according to the blood of each that is put in. As examples of this the Halfbred sheep (between Border Leicester and Cheviot), the Corriedale (a halfbred between Lincoln and Merino) and the Polwarth (a back cross of the Corriedale to the Merino) may be mentioned. However, it will be realized from what has been said above that, where the breeds crossed differ materially in the unit-factor segregating characters (such as colour, horns and patterns), a large number of different types may arise when the second generation is bred. To eliminate the unwanted ones rigorous selection is necessary. Therefore large numbers of animals to choose from is an essential starting point in any programme of breed transformation.

In the U.S.A., a new red bacon pig, the Minnesota No. 1, has been produced by crossing the while Danish Landrace having good bacon qualities with the red Canadian Tamworth. Boars which had good bacon qualities and red colour in the second generation were progeny tested and those which bred true were used to form the new breed. Much the same process was followed in forming a new breed of cattle, the Santa Gertrudis, to combine the beef qualities of the Shorthorn with the heat-resisting qualities of Zebu cattle. A bull was found by progeny testing which bred true for the characters desired and he was linebred to form the new breed. Experiments are now being made in India and Australia to produce, in the same way, a new dairy bred of cattle suitable for the tropics by crossing European dairy breeds with the Indian Zebu.

5

Nuclear Transplantation in Cow and Buffalo

Nuclear transfer (NT) is one of the most interesting and challenging areas of science to emerge in recent years. It is a technique that goes back to early experiments in the frog, *Rana pipiens*, and in the toad, *Xenopus leavis*. The principle of the enucleated egg reprogramming the donor cell to produce identical offspring was continued in mammals. This technique relied on the use of early embryos as the donor of the nucleus. As the early embryos used were pre-compacted, with 16–32 cells, the number of cells available for the production of cloned animals was limited, although many animals were produced by this method. The next step was to produce animals from the *inner cell mass* (ICM) of the blastocyst, but there was still a shortage of cells with which to make clones. One of the greatest breakthroughs was production of a cell line from thc ICM. This made possible the production of millions of identical cells for the procedure, allowing the production of many identical clones, the cryopreservation of cells for storage, and the potential for the cells to be genetically modified. The story carries on through the birth of Dolly, the first animal cloned from an adult cell, in 1996 to the present day, with many animals having now been born all over the world by this technique. Animals successfully cloned so far include sheep, cattle, goats, mice, pigs, rabbits and, most recently, cats, although considerable efforts are being made towards the cloning of other species. One recent advance is in the cloning of rare and endangered species such as the Gaur, Mouflon and Enderby Island cattle breed. The success rate of NT consistently falls within the range of 1–5%, showing that, at the moment, the technique has an inherent inefficiency. There are many theories as to the reason for this inefficiency but, at present, these remain speculative. Embryos transferred to surrogate mothers are lost in an unusual pattern in NT, as losses can occur throughout pregnancy and continue after parturition. There have also been defects in many of the animals produced from NT, with reports of animals with defective immune systems, cardiovascular problems, obesity, urogenital abnormalities, and many more problems, many of which are fatal. Dolly herself suffered from arthritis but no one knows whether this was due to the NT process or a chance event in her life.

However, the possible benefits of NT are very great. In particular, the expansion in the number of the available techniques with which to make precise genetic changes in animals by gene targeting in the donor cells, creates many new opportunities in biology, medicine and agriculture. This approach was used to insert genes that direct production of proteins in the milk of livestock, and has since been used to delete a gene from pigs with the aim of being able to use the organs for transplantation into human patients. Genetic selection of the nuclear donor leads to production of genetically modified clones of the desired gender and appropriate production traits. The purpose of this chapter is to give details of procedures that have been used in our laboratory.

Tools and Equipment

Micromanipulation

An inverted Nikon Eclipse TE300 with differential interference contrast optics and epi-fluorescence is used. This microscope is equipped with 4X, 10X, 20X phase contrast, and 40X DIC lenses and 10X eyepieces. The microscope is fitted with a long working distance condenser, which allows extra room to work on the microscope stage. It is fitted with two Narishige MO-188NE three-dimensional hydraulic oil micromanipulators, which are of the hanging joystick type. Two Narishige microinjectors of model IM-16 or IM-188 are used, these being fitted with either a 250 μl gas-tight Hamilton syringe for the holding side of the micro tools or a 100 μl gas-tight Hamilton syringe for the enucleation side. These microinjectors are fitted with a three-way stop-cock (Vigon VG1) and a 5 ml syringe to allow the hydraulic system to be filled easily without having to dismantle the system. The system is filled with Fluorinert (FC77), which is an inert hydraulic fluid, take care to eliminate any air bubbles from the system, as these act like a spring making the injectors difficult to control. The microinjectors are connected to tool holders by polytetrafluoroethylene (PTFE) tubing, the left injector controlling the right tool and the right injector controlling the left tool. This system allows both movement of the joystick and manipulation of the suction on the micro tool to be controlled simultaneously.

Microtools

Glass microtools for the oocyte-holding pipette are either purchased from Humagen or can be custom made as follows. The holding pipette is made by pulling a 1 mm glass capillary over a small Bunsen flame to give an outside diameter of 150 μm. The pipette is then bent and the end fire-polished to give an internal diameter of 20 μm, which will allow it to enter horizontally into the manipulation chamber. The enucleation pipette is straight with a long taper and a bevel of 35° and spike, with an external diameter of around 18 μm.

Manipulation Chamber

The manipulation chamber is made by taking a sterile, good quality, siliconized glass slide and placing two strips of sterile glass, 2 × 5 × 25 mm, on the slide, sealing the strip down with petroleum jelly (Vaseline Ponds) to make it liquid tight, then applying a little petroleum jelly on the upper surface of the glass strips. A 300 pl drop of manipulation medium (hSOF - Ca +FCS) is then placed between the glass strips and a clean sterile glass coverslip is placed on the top, making a liquid-tight seal with the petroleum jelly. The ends of the chamber are then sealed with mineral oil to make a liquid-tight

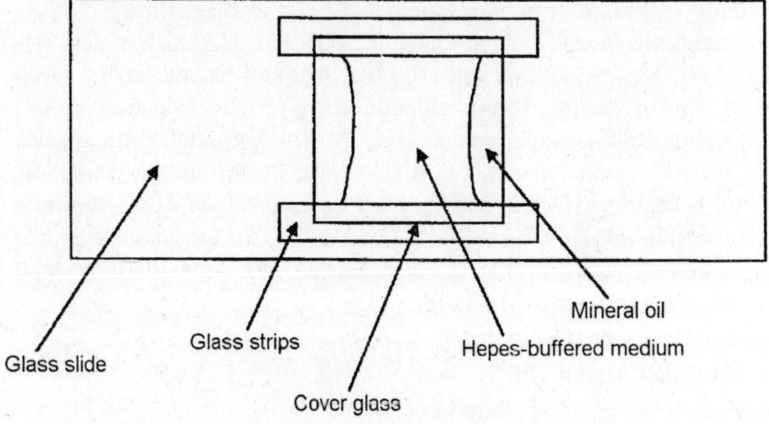

Fig. 5.1. Manipulation chamber.

chamber, which will maintain the osmolarity of the solution in the chamber. The manipulation chamber can then be placed on the microscope stage and the glass microtools inserted from either side. Oocytes or cells can be inserted into the chamber using a small glass capillary, which is pushed through the oil.

Oocyte Handling

Oocytes are handled on Leica Mz 7.5 or Mz 12.5 dissecting microscopes with Linkum MS 100 warm stages or Mini Tub HT 200 temperature control units. The temperature is held at 37°C.

Cell Fusion

Cells are fused with a BSL CF-150 cell fusion device. This is connected to a custom-made fusion chamber consisting of two platinum electrodes, which are stuck to the bottom of a glass Petri dish with epoxy resin adhesive (Araldite), at a distance of 200 μm apart.

Embryo Culture

NT embryos are cultured in a Heraeus BB6060 triple gas incubator with a gas mixture of 5% O_2, 5% CO_2, 90% N_2, at 39°C in a humidified atmosphere.

Supplies

All chemicals (and catalogue numbers) are from Sigma, unless stated otherwise.

1. Fluorinert FC 77 (F-4758); $NaHCO_3$ (S-5761); Phenol Red (P-5530); pyruvic acid (P-4562); $CaCl_2 \cdot 2H_2O$ (C-7902); glucose (G-6152); $MgCl_2 \cdot 6H_2O$ (M-2393); NaCl(S-5886); KCl (P-5405); KH_2PO_4 (P-5655); kanamycin sulphate (K-1377); Penicillin (P-7794); Streptomycin (S-1277); L-glutamine (G5763); Hepes, free acid (H-6147); Hepes, sodium salt (H-3784); sodium lactate (60%) syrup (L-7900); bovine serum albumin (BSA), fatty-acid-free (FAF) (A8806); non essential amino acids (M-7145); essential amino acids (B-6766); cytochalasin B (CB; C-6762); hyaluronidase (H-3884); bis benzimide (Hoechst 33342; B-2261); mannitol (M-4125), dimethyl sulfoxide (DMSO; D-4540), Sigmacote (SL-2); estradiol (E-2758); leutinizing hormone (LH; L-5269); $MgSO_4 \cdot 7H_2O$ (M-1880); mineral oil, embryo tested (M-8410)
2. TCM199 with Earles Salts
3. Fetal calf serum (FCS)
4. Follicle stimulating hormone (FSH)
5. 18 μm bevelled and sharpened pipettes. Humagen

Media and Solutions

Aspiration Medium

1. Hepes-buffered TCM 199
2. 10% FCS, heat inactivated

Dissection Medium (50 ml)

1. 45 ml TCM 199 with Earles salts (Gibco)
2. 75.0 mg/l kanamycin monosulfate
3. 7.08 g/l Hepes (pH 7.8 osmolarity 279 mosmol/kg H_2O)
4. 5 ml FCS (heat inactivated)

Maturation Medium

For 10 ml:

1. 8.89 ml Bicarbonate-buffered TCM199
2. 1 ml FCS
3. 0.1 ml LH stock (1 μg/ml final concentration)
4. 0.1 IU FSH (Ovagen) 0.9 mg
5. Filter sterilize then add
6. 0.01 ml estradiol (1 μg/ml final concentration)
7. Equilibrate at 39°C in 5% CO_2 for 2 h
8. Add 0.1 ml 10 mM cysteamine (make up weekly and store at 4°C)

Stock Solution B (250 mM $NaHCO_3$)

1. 1.05 g $NaHCO_3$
2. Phenol Red (2–3 grains)
3. Make up to 50 ml with MilliQ dH_2O (Osmolarity 430–440)
4. Store filtered at 4°C for 3 weeks

Stock Solution C (33 mM pyruvate)

1. 0.036 g pyruvic acid
2. Make up to 10 ml with MilliQ dH_2O (Osmolarity 55–60)
3. Store filtered at 4°C for 1 week

Stock Solution D (171 mM $CaCl_2$ $2H_2O$)

1. 1.26 g $CaCl_2 \cdot 2H_2O$
2. Make up to 50 ml with MilliQ dH_2O
3. Osmolarity 430–440
4. Store filtered at 4°C for 3 months

Stock Solution G (60 mM Glucose)

1. 0.54 g glucose

2. Make up to 50 ml with MilliQ dH_2O
3. Store filtered at 4°C
4. Osmolarity 60–70
5. Store filtered at 4°C for 3 months

Stock Solution GLN (10 mM L-Glutamine)

1. 0.0438 g L-Glutamine
2. Make upto 30 ml with dH_2O
3. Store filtered at 4°C for 1 week

Stock Solution H (250 mM Hepes)

1. 3.0 g Hepes (free acid)
2. 3.25 g Hepes (sodium salt)
3. Phenol Red (2–3 grains)
4. Make up to 100 ml with MilliQ dH_2O
5. Osmolarity 380–385
6. Store filtered at 4°C for 1 month

Stock Solution K (kanamycin sulphate)

1. 0.5 g kanamycin sulphate
2. Make up to 10 ml with MilliQ dH_2O
3. Store filtered at 4°C for 3 months
4. Dilute 1:1,000 for a final concentration of 50 μg/ml

Stock Solution L (330 mM Na lactate)

1. 11.75 ml Na lactate (60%) syrup
2. Make up to 250 ml with MilliQ dH_2O
3. Osmolarity 590–640
4. Store filtered at 4°C for 3 months

Stock Solution M ($MgCl_2 \cdot 6H_2O$)

1. 2.0 g $MgCl_2 \cdot 6H_2O$
2. Make up to 200 ml with MilliQ dH_2O
3. Osmolarity 120–130
4. Store filtered at 4°C for 3 months

Stock Solution S2

1. 6.29 g NaCl
2. 0.534 g KCl
3. 0.162 g KH_2PO_4
4. 0.025 g Kanamycin (or 0.06 g Penicillin + 0.05 g Streptomycin)
5. Make up to 100 ml with MilliQ dH_2O

6. Osmolarity 2173
7. Store filtered at 4°C for 3 months

Hepes Synthetic Oviduct Fluid (hSOF) +Ca

	To make 100 ml
Stock 2	10.0 ml
Stock B	0.2 ml
Stock H	8.0 ml
Stock C	1.0 ml
Stock D	1.0 ml
Stock M	1.0 ml
Stock L	1.0 ml
Stock G	2.5 ml
MilliQ H_2O	73.5 ml

1. Osmolarity 265–275
2. pH 7.4
3. Add 0.3 g BSA (FAF)
4. Filter and store at 4°C for 1–2 weeks

Hepes SOF (hSOF) –Ca

	To make 100 ml
Stock 2	10.0 ml
Stock B	2.0 ml
Stock H	8.0 ml
Stock C	1.0 ml
Stock M	1.0 ml
Stock L	1.0 ml
Stock G	2.5 ml
MilliQ H_2O	74.5 ml

1. Osmolarity 265–275
2. pH 7.4
3. Add 0.3 g BSA (FAF)
4. Filter and store at 4°C for 1–2 weeks

Culture Medium (SOFaaBSA)

	To make 100 ml
Stock 2	10.0 ml
Stock B	10.0 ml
Stock C	1.0 ml

Stock D	1.0 ml
Stock M	1.0 ml
Stock L	1.0 ml
Stock G	2.5 ml
Stock GLN	10.0 ml
Non essential amino acids	1.0 ml
Essential amino acids	2.0 ml
MilliQ H_2O	60.5 ml

1. Osmolarity 265–275
2. pH 7.4
3. Add 0.8 g BSA (FAF)
4. Filter and store at 4°C for 1 week

Fusion Medium

1. Mannitol 0.3 M
2. $MgSO_4 \cdot 7H_2O$ 0.1 mM
3. $CaCl_2 \cdot 2H_2O$ 0.05 mM
4. Filter and store at –20°C
5. Note: Use a 0.2 μm syringe filter

PROCEDURE

Oocyte Maturation

Reagents required:

- PBS
- Dissection medium
- FCS
- Maturation medium
- Oil

1. Oocytes are prepared by collection of ovaries in a warm container following slaughter of heifers.
2. The ovaries are transported to the laboratory, in warm PBS, within 4 h of slaughter and should be between 25 and 35°C when they reach the laboratory.
3. The ovaries are thoroughly washed in warm saline to remove excess blood before follicles are aspirated with an 18-gauge needle and 10 ml syringe. Note. Only follicles between 4 and 8 mm should be selected for aspiration.
4. The follicles are pierced and the cumulus oocyte complexes (COCs) removed in the follicular fluid by applying gentle suction on the

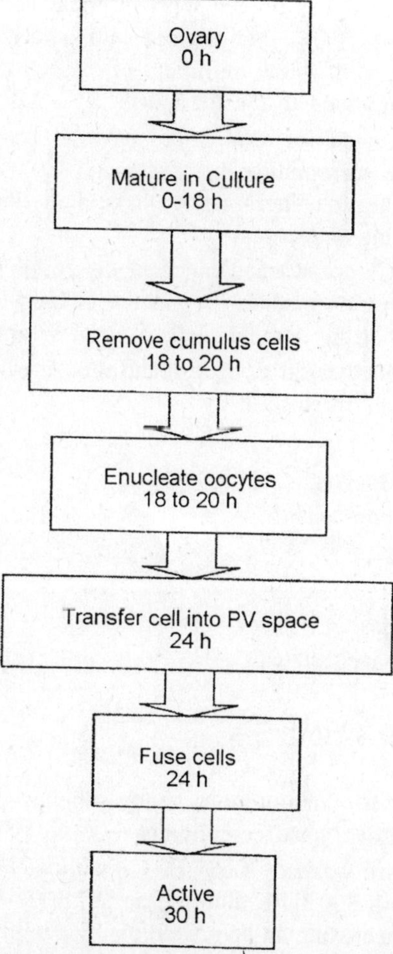

Fig. 5.2. Schematic representation of nuclear transfer (NT) procedure.

piston of the syringe. Each follicle contains one COC, and the number of follicles per ovary is variable, some producing one or two and others up to four or five.

5. The aspirated follicular fluid containing the COCs is gently expelled into a universal tube and kept warm in a water bath until the ovaries have been aspirated.
6. The COCs are allowed to settle for 10 min before the excess follicular fluid is carefully aspirated from the top of the tube using a sterile plastic pipette.

7. The follicular fluid is diluted with an equal volume of dissection medium +10% FCS, then poured into a large Petri dish. The tube is rinsed with a few milliliters of dissection medium +FCS, which is then added to the Petri dish.
8. A search is made for COCs that have at least three layers of cumulus cells surrounding the oocyte. COCs with fewer cumulus cells are either degenerating or have had the cells physically removed during collection.
9. Selected COCs are washed twice in dissection medium and then once in maturation medium. A pipettor is used to move the media around, so that the cumulus cells are not scraped off.
10. Culture ten oocytes/50 μl drop maturation medium under oil in a 5% CO_2 in air mixture at 39°.

8.4.2

Enucleation of Oocytes

Reagents required:

- hSOF –Ca
- FCS
- Hyaluronidase
- Nunc four-well plates
- CB
- Hoechst 33342 dye
- BSA (FAF)

1. After 18–20 h of maturation, gently pipette up and down a few times to remove any free cumulus.
2. The COCs are washed in hSOF –Ca without FCS before transfer to a well with 300 IU hyaluronidase in hSOF –Ca –FCS and then gently pipetted using an automatic pipettor until all of the cumulus cells have been removed. A 100 or 200 μl volume is sucked into the pipette from a 500 μl volume in a Nunc four-well plate. Keep the pipette at an angle so as the oocytes are not damaged by being squeezed against the bottom or side of the well.
3. Wash in hSOF –Ca +10% FCS.
4. Oocytes with a first polar body are selected under a dissecting microscope by gently rolling the oocytes until the polar body is seen. These oocytes, which are thought to be mature and at MII, are then stored in hSOF –Ca +10% FCS in a warm box at 37°C until required.

5. Oocytes put to one side as not having a polar body can be examined again later.
6. Batches of 10–15 oocytes are placed in hSOF -Ca plus 7.5 μg/ml CB and 10 μg/ml Hoechst 33342 for 15 min prior to enucleation.
7. Oocytes are placed in the manipulation chamber with hSOF -Ca +FCS with CB.
8. Move the holding pipette to the oocyte and apply gentle suction until an oocyte is picked up.
9. This oocyte is then raised above the rest of the oocytes, and the microscope stage moved to an area of the chamber away from any other oocytes.
10. Turn the oocyte using the enucleation pipette until the polar body is in a position where the pipette can be pushed through the zona pellucida, the polar body and the adjacent cytoplasm within the body of the oocyte (where the metaphase plate is located), such that the polar body and metaphase plate can be aspirated gently into the pipette. An 18 μm pipette ground at 35° with a pipette beveller and a spike put on the end with a hot glass bead on a microforge to allow it to go easily through the zona pellucida, is used.
11. The holding pipette with oocyte attached is removed from the field of view; the white light is turned off before the enucleation pipette is exposed to UV light. The DNA in the polar body will be seen to fluoresce brightly, with the maternal DNA fluorescing less brightly. Depending on the orientation of the metaphase plate, the chromosomes can be seen as circular, linear or any configuration in between. *Note:* it is important that the enucleated oocyte is not exposed to UV light.
12. Successfully enucleated oocytes are deposited to the right of the chamber so that they can be easily removed, using a small hand-drawn glass pipette.
13. Wash enucleated oocytes in hSOF -Ca +FCS. Store in the incubator in SOF -Ca +BSA (0.8 mg/ml FAF BSA). *Note:* enucleation of the oocyte is most easily carried out as soon as the polar body is expelled, as the metaphase lies near the polar body at this time. Therefore the polar body can be used as a marker for enucleation. Polar bodies are expelled from around 18 h of maturation onwards, so enucleation can begin at around 20 h post maturation. Electrofusion can then be carried out at 24 h.

Cell Preparation

Reagents required:

- Donor cell culture medium
- Trypsin
- hSOF
- FCS

1. Donor cells are prepared by serum starving cells in culture before they reach confluence by reducing the serum from 10% to 0.5% for 5 days. This causes the majority of the cells to enter quiescence (G0). (*Note:* cells used for NT have often been serum starved to induce quiescence and this enhances the efficiency of the procedure. Allowing the cells to become confluent may also aid efficiency, since this also results in cell quiescence)
2. The cells are trypsinized until they are in a single cell suspension, and then washed and re-suspended in hSOF +0.5% FCS medium until injection.

Injection of Cells

Reagents required:

- hSOF –Ca
- FAF BSA

1. Cells are transferred to the top right-hand corner of a fresh manipulation chamber with hSOF –CA +BSA (0:8 mg/ml FAF BSA).
2. Batches often enucleated oocytes are transferred to the center of the chamber using a small hand-drawn pipette.
3. Oocytes are picked up using the holding pipette.
4. A number of cells are then picked up in the injection pipette and a single intact cell is injected through the zona pellucida and into the perivitelline space of each of the enucleated oocytes. Care must be taken to ensure that the cell is alive and is making good contact with the oocyte cytoplasm for fusion to take place. Live cells have a bright shiny cell membrane, but if they lyse during cell transfer, the cell membrane becomes dull.

Electrofusion

Reagents required:

- Fusion medium
- hSOF –Ca
- FCS

- FAF BSA
- oil

1. The couplets are removed from the manipulation chamber, washed in fusion medium, and placed in the fusion chamber.
2. The couplets are all placed to one side of the electrodes, and each couplet is lifted in turn, using a small glass pipette, and placed between the electrodes.
3. Couplets are manually aligned so that the point of contact between the cell and oocyte is parallel to the electrodes. Precise orientation of the couplet is required for fusion to take place.
4. An alternating current (AC) current of 0.25 kV/cm is applied for a period of 5 s, and followed by 3× direct current (DC) pulses of 1.25 kV/cm of 80 μs in rapid succession.
5. Couplets are removed from the fusion chamber and deposited in a wash dish containing hSOF –Ca +FCS.
6. Upon completion of this procedure, the batch of couplets are removed from the wash and transferred to 30 μl drops of SOF – Ca +BSA under oil and incubated at 39°C in 5% CO_2 in air.
7. Check if fusion has taken place after 1 h.
8. Up to 100 oocytes can be handled comfortably each manipulation day.

Activation

Reagents required:

- hSOF+Ca
- FAF BSA
- Ionomycin
- SOFaaBSA
- 6-dimethylaminopurine

1. 30 min before activation wash in hSOF +Ca + BSA (1 mg/ml FAF BSA)
2. At 26–30 h post-maturation, the embryos are activated by placing them in hSOF +Ca +BSA containing 5 μM ionomycin at room temperature for 5 min.
3. The embryos are repeatedly washed in hSOF +Ca +BSA (30 mg/ml FAF BSA) to remove the ionomycin.
4. Culture for 4 h in SOFaaBSA (0.8 mg/ml FAF BSA) with 2 mM 6-dimethylaminopurine (6-DMAP) at 39°C in a 5% O_2:5% CO_2:90% N_2 gas mixture in drops under oil.

5. Wash in pre-gassed SOFaaBSA (0.8 mg/ml FAF BSA)
6. Culture until the blastocyst stage is reached.

Culture

Reagents required:

- SOFaa
- FAF BSA

1. The successfully fused and activated embryos are transferred to 500 μl SOFaa+BSA, overlaid with mineral oil, in Nunc four-well plates at 39°C in a 5% O_2:5% CO_2:90% N_2 gas mixture.
2. Embryos should have developed to become blastocysts on day 7 of culture. *Note:* The success of NT is dependent on a large numbers of variables, from the treatment of the heifers prior to slaughter, to the "cell line", which is used as the nuclear donor, so it is very difficult to give accurate figures for the success of the procedure.

Cloning statistics

1. 14–69% reach morula/blastocyst stage, as a percentage of embryos enucleated and reconstructed.
2. 0–100% pregnant, as a percentage of the number of pregnancies detected to the number of recipient animals.
3. 0–83% live births, as a percentage of embryos transferred.
4. 0–2.8% cloning efficiency, as a percentage of live offspring from those enucleated and reconstructed.

Troubleshooting

As mentioned earlier, NT is a procedure involving a great many steps, many of which are critical to the success of the technique. Oocyte quality is very important, and it is wise to incorporate some controls into the procedure to make sure that the oocytes are of good quality and that they are at the correct stage of development. This is the rationale behind selecting oocytes with polar bodies, as these are liable to be at the MII stage.

It may also be wise to make sure that the oocytes are at the correct stage for activation by activating a sample at different times following maturation.

Routine maintenance of equipment and recording of temperatures and gas concentrations of incubators can prevent problems.

Make sure that the holding pipette is lifted above the level of the other oocytes when moving the pipette around as it can easily move the other oocytes in the chamber if it is not lifted high enough. The area where enucleation is carried out should be a sufficient distance from the other oocytes and the enucleated oocyte on the holding pipette, to ensure that only the enucleation pipette is exposed to UV radiation.

When transferring cells to the perivitelline space of the enucleated oocyte, care must be taken to ensure that the cytoplasm and cell are in contact, so that electrofusion can take place.

If using cultured cells, karyotype the cell line at regular intervals to make sure that the cells have not developed an abnormal karyotype during culture.

Different cells require different periods of serum starvation to trigger quiescence, and this can be determined by proliferating cell nuclear antigen (PCNA) staining. PCNA is a nuclear antigen visible during S-phase of the cell cycle.

Buffalo

The domestic buffalo or water buffalo belongs to the *Bovidae* family and from time immemorial has been a domestic animal in India, Malaya and Egypt. It occupies an important place amongst the domestic animals of the tropics as a provider of dairy produce, beef and draught power. Its greatest asset as a domestic animal is its ability to subsist on the coarsest fodder and to convert it most efficiently into animal produce.

The water buffalo is found in a more or less domesticated state throughout the northern tropical and sub-tropical zones in Asia as well as in the Philippines and Trinidad and in all countries of the Mediterranean basin except France. In the southern tropical zone it is found in Indonesia and it has been introduced to Melville Island near the northern coast of Australia. It is also found wild in the Northern Territories of Australia but the original animals were domesticated.

In recent years, the buffalo commonly known as an 'Asian Animal' has attracted global concern. The buffalo is the dairy, draught and meat animal of Asia. The Indian subcontinent is the home tract of the world's dairy buffaloes. To-day in India, the water buffalo is recognized as her milk machine. It accounts for more than half of India's total milk production, although it constitutes only one third of the total milch population. Nevertheless, its potential for milk production remains only partially tapped, as almost 80 to 85 per cent buffaloes are non-descript, yielding on an average no more than 1.5 litres of milk per day in contrast to an average of 7 to 8 litres of daily milk yield obtained from well bred milch breeds.

The domesticated buffaloes may be classified into two main categories, viz., (1) the swamp buffalo (chromosomes, 2n = 48) and (2) the river buffalo (chromosomes, 2n = 50). They belong to the same species, *Bubalus bubalis* but have very different habits.

Some Common Terms in Relation to Buffalo

Details	*Expressions*
Species called as	Bovine of Butaline
Group of animals	Herd
Adult male	Buffalo bull
Adult female	She-buffalo or buffalo cow
Young male	Buffalo bull calf
Young female	Buffalo heifer calf
New-born one	Buffalo calf
Castrated male	Buffalo Bullock
Castrated female	Spayed
Female with its offspring	Calf at foot
Act of parturition	Calving
Act of mating	Serving
Sound produced	Bellowing
Pregnancy	Gestation

As the name implies, the water buffalo, whether of the river or the swamp type, has an inherent predilection for water and loves wallowing in water or mud pools. The river buffaloes, as a rule, shows preference for clean running water, whereas the swamp buffalo likes to wallow in mudholes, swamps and stagnant pools. Like cattle buffaloes are good swimmer. The river and swamp buffaloes vary slightly in body structure, size and colour. A swamp buffalo is recognised by its short stocky body, short face with wide muzzle and short thin legs. These buffaloes are usually dark grey in colour, although variations from black to albinoids are found among the population. Swamp buffaloes vary in size from 300 to 600 kilograms. They are primarily used as draught animals, but they do provide small quantities of milk for a farmer's family.

Breeds of Indian Buffaloes

Only in India are there found well-defined tropical breeds with standard qualities and, even there, well-bred individuals are far out numbered by nondescript animals. In other countries, although distinct types are to be found, no type has the specific physical characters which mark it from other types so that it can be unquestionably recognized.

Good, well-defined, milk breeds are found only in the Punjab, Rajasthan, and the Gujarat district of Bombay, but in Central and South India there is a noted draught breed.

These animals belong to a non-descript class and these vary greatly in size, weight and general features known as *deshi*. However, on the basis of regions the well defined buffalo breeds are as follows:

Table 5.1

Murrah Group	*Gujarat Group*	*Uttar Pradesh Group*	*Central India Group*	*South India Group*
Murrah	Surti	Bhadawari	Nagpuri	Toda
Nili-Ravi	Jaffarbadi	Tarai	Pandhepuri	South Kanara
Kundi	Mehsana		Manda	
Godavari			Jerangi	
			Kalhandi	
			Sambalpur	

Murrah

The *Murrah* is the most important Indian breed of buffalo, and is the most efficient producer of milk, not only in India but probably in the world. Bulls of this breed are used extensively for up-grading inferior stock. She-buffaloes are used in most of the important cities for the supply of milk and ghee. The home of the breed is mainly in Punjab and Delhi, but animals are bred pure in the United Provinces, Rajasthan and other places. Rohtak in Punjab is a well-known market from where thousands of high yielders are exported.

The Murrah has a deep massive frame with short, broad back and a comparatively light neck and head. It has short, characteristics tightly curled horns, well-developed udder and long tail with a white switch reaching to the fetlock. Other features are: short massive limbs with good bone, broad hoofs and drooping quarters. The colour is usually black, but fawn-grey colouring of the hair and white markings on the face, legs or tail are not uncommon. 'Wall' eyes are also not unusual.

The skin is soft, smooth with scanty hair. The body weight of bulls amounts on the average to 550 kg that of the she-buffaloes to 450 kg. The height at withers on the average is 1.42 m for bulls and 1.32 m for she-buffaloes.

Production

The average milking capacity in established herds is about 1400 to 2000 kg with a butter fat content of 7 per cent of milk in a lactation of 9 to 10 months.

Nili/Ravi

The *Nili* and *Ravi* are two types of buffaloes found in the valley of the rivers Sutlej and Ravi in the Districts of Montgomery and Ferozepur. There is no essential difference between the two types although for a long time they were treated as different breeds, but closer study indicated that it was a distinction without a difference, and now they are officially treated as one breed.

This is considered to be one of the best breeds of buffaloes in India, next only to the Murrah. Like the Murrah large numbers are exported annually from the breeding areas for milk production in cities. The average milk yield is practically the same as that of the Murrah.

These animals have a medium-sized, deep frame with an elongated, coarse and heavy head, bulging at the top, depressed between the eyes and ending in a fine muzzle. Horns are small with a high coil and the neck is long, thin and fine. It is the face and forehead that distinguish this breed mainly from the Murrah.

The typical Nili/Ravi cow has a well-developed udder. The tail is long, almost touching the ground.

The colour is usually black, but brown is not uncommon. Pink markings are sometimes seen on the udder and brisket. White markings on the forehead, face, muzzle and legs, white switch and wall, eyes, which are also seen, are much liked by breeders. The average live-weight and measurements of mature animals are as follows:

	Male	*Female*
Live-weight : pounds (kg.)	1,300 (589.7)	1,000 (453.6)
Height at withers : inches (cm.)	54.0 (137.2)	53.5 (135.9)
Length from point of shoulder to pin Bone : inches (cm.)	62.5 (158.8)	58.5 (148.6)

Surti

The *Surti* is a popular breed found in the 'Charottar' tract of Gujarat in Mumbai State between Mahi and Sabarmati rivers. The

Surti is known to be an economic milk producer and the average lactation yield is reported to be 3,650 pounds (1,655.5 kg.) milk with 7.5 per cent fat.

Surti buffaloes are well-shaped animals of medium size. They are rather low on the legs and have a mild and placid disposition, but the general appearance is bright, with prominent, round, rather bulging eyes. The horns are of medium length and are sickle-shaped. The colour is black or brown; good specimens have two white collars, one just round the jowl from ear to ear and a second lower down around the brisket akin to the breast plate worn by horses. No other breed of buffalo has as straight a back as this one. The udder is well shaped and well developed with pinkish-coloured skin and medium-sized teats, placed squarely. The skin is fairly thick but pliable, soft and smooth, with scanty hair.

The average measurements of mature animals are as follows:

	Male	*Female*
Height at withers : inches (cm.)	51.5 (130.8)	49.0 (124.5)
Length from point of shoulder to pin Bone: inches (cm.)	56.3 (154.2)	54.5 (138.4)

Jaffarabadi

Jaffarabadi buffaloes are very massive animals and are seen in their purest from in the Gir forest of Kathiawar where they are bred in large numbers, almost solely for ghee production. They consume large quantities of fodder but the milk yield is high and the butterfat content exceptionally high. Their noticeable feature is the very prominent forehead and heavy horns which are inclined to droop on each side of the neck and then turn up at the points but not in such a tight curl as in Murrah buffaloes. They are usually black in colour.

Mehsana

This breed is found in districts of Bombay State and neighbouring areas. It is considered to be an intermediate type between Surti and Murrah buffaloes but here is a considerable amount of variation from one district to another. The horns of these animals are usually curled after the manner of Murrah buffaloes but not so tightly. They are either black or fawn-grey in colour with usually some white marking on the face, legs, or tip of the tail. The udder is usually well shaped with uniformly placed teats. Mehsana buffaloes are considered to be particularly valuable milch cattle because of their early maturity, persistence in milk production and regularity in breeding. They are of medium size, economical to feed, and are used largely for milk and ghee production in Bombay state.

Uttar Pradesh Group

Bhadawari

Bhadawari estate of Agra district and adjoining areas of Gwalior and Etawah. Animals are found scattered in the surroundings of Jamuna and Chambal rivers.

Medium size and wedge-shaped body. Comparatively small head bulging towards horms. Legs are short but stout. Hooves of the hind quarters are more backward than fore quarters. Colour is copper, hair scanty. Barrel is short but well developed.

Table 5.2

Trait	*Range of vale*
Age at first calving (months)	48.3—50.78
Lactation yield (lit.)	1111—1252
Lactation length (days)	276
Calving interval (days)	453.6
Dry period	156

Forehead is slightly broad and deep in the middle. Face is comparatively narrow with slightly marked nose. Eyes are prominent, active and bright. Udder is not so well developed but milk veins are fairly prominent. Teats are of medium size and uniform in length.

Average yield ranges from 2,000 to 2,070 kg. in a lactation period of 305 days with a high fat percentage. Males are used for draught purposes.

Tarai

The breed gets the name from the *Tarai* area of U.P., where it is mostly found between Tanakpur and Ramnagar. The breed is native to hilly area. They are frequently crossed with Murrah bulls.

It has a moderate body, slightly convex head with prominent nasal bones. Horns are long and flat with coils, bending backwards and upwards having pointed tips. The eyes are rather small but ears are long and coarse. Legs are short but strong. The tail is long, reaching below the hocks. The colour of the skin varies from black to brown. Sometimes there is a white blaze on the forehead. The switch of the tail is white.

The breed is poor regarding milk production, which may be as low as 2-3 kg daily. Males are efficient draught animals used for agricultural operations as powers including transport. Tarai breed is well adapted to the difficult environmental situations and nutritional conditions of the Tarai.

Central India Group

Nagpuri

Synonym, Marathwada, Berari, Ellichpuri, Gaulani, Varad, Gauli.

As the name applies, these animals are mostly found in Nagpur including Wardha, Yeotmal, Akola, Buldana, Amrawati and Achalpur in Maharastra. The breed has got several strains differing in colour and other superficial traits.

The colour is usually black; occasionally white markings are observed on the face, legs and switch. In general the breed is known as lighter type than those of north, not so squat and have a short tail. The face is long and thin with a straight profile. The neck is also longer with heavy brisket. It has long horns flat-curved reaches towards back over the shoulders. Naval flap is short or almost absent.

Male body weight averages 525 kg. while female attains about 425 kg. The average height at withers in male 142 cm and that of cows 132 cm; heart girth is 210 and 205 cm. for male and female respectively. The females are moderately good yielders, producing on an average 1,000 litres milk per lactation of 300 days with butter fat content between 7.0-8.5 per cent. The males are used for heavy draught but are slow.

Pandhepuri

Synonym Pandharpur, Dharwari

The breed is widely distributed in south Maharastra, parts of Andhra Pradesh and Karnataka States.

Animals are of medium size with long narrow face and very long, flat and usually twisted thin horns.

Males are hardy and well suited for drought purpose.

Manda

Synonym, Parlakimedi, Ganjam.

The animals are bred in the hills above Parlakimedi and Mandasa on the borders of Orissa and Andhra Pradesh. Basically the breed is reared in areas of thick forest usually on natural herbage and brought down to the plains for sale.

The general colour is brown or grey with yellowish tufts of hair on the knees and fetlocks, and the switch is yellowish white. The breed is a medium sized animal. The eyes are sharp with a broad red margin around the lids. The horns are broad and semi-circular extending backward and inward. The forehead is flat with short muzzle. Neck and forelegs are also short but stout with well developed chest.

Milk yield is satisfactory. Males are hardy and like a bullock can work in the hot sun. It can draw a load of about a ton but at a slow pace.

Sambalpur

Synonyms, Kimedi, Gowdoo.

The home tract of this breed is controversial. Originally it was known to be habitat of Sambalpur area of Orissa, later on it has been suggested that the main habitat of this breed is around Bilaspur district of Madhya Pradesh wherefrom calves are brought by 'gowdoo' (Herdman) to Sambalpur area.

Animals are large and powerful having long, narrow barrel and prominent fore-head. Body and coat colour is generally black but it varies to brown and ash grey.

Males are very active and good for drought purposes which are affected by high atmosphere temperature. Females breed regularly and produce milk satisfactorily.

Kalhandi

Synonym, Peddakimedi.

The home tract of this breed has been referred to the eastern part of Andhra Pradesh and adjoining areas of Orissa.

A strong with broad horns and half curved running backward at the tip. Body colour is between grey and ash grey. It has well developed chest and strong fore-limbs. Eyes are prominent and large with narrow red margin around the lids. Tail is of medium length with white switch. Due to light colour it tolerates heat more than dark coloured buffaloes.

Animals are docile and hardy. They are used to carry loads in hilly areas as well as for ploughing in plains. Milk yield is satisfactory.

Jerangi

This breed of buffalo is widely distributed in Jerangi hills of Orissa and northern parts of Visakhapatnam and west of Ganjam in Andhra Pradesh, One of the dwarf breeds of buffalo and its height does not exceed four feet. Horns are conical and small, and run backward, body colour is black.

Not that much good in milk production but are useful animals for ploughing in water-logged paddy fields.

South India Group

Toda

The name of the breed originates from the name of *Toda* tribes of Nilgiri hills of Tamil Nadu State who rear this breed.

These are large-sized animals having long barrel and strong build. Horns of these buffaloes are variable in shape but are usually set wide apart run outward, upward and then inward at the top. Face is short and wide. Hump and dewlap are absent, chest is broad and deep; legs are short and sturdy. Along the crest of the neck, hump area and back, there is a thick growth of hair like a mane which imparts a bison like appearance.

The animals are not always docile. All of sudden they may become furious and dangerous particularly to unknown persons. When necessary, they fight against even tigers and other wild animals in an organised team.

Females are good milkers, yields between 4.5-8.5 litres daily with an average of 7.0% fat and possesses typical well-flavoured taste.

Breeding and Management Problems

Buffaloes are Seasonal Breeders

In tropical countries like India, *she* buffaloes indicate seasonal sex periodicity in respect of oestrous and conception. As much as 62.8% animals show periodicity in October to February with the peak around December and this period coincides with higher conception rate. During the period from March to September, with comparatively longer days and higher intensity of sun, ovarian activity appears to be adversely affected.

Buffalo bulls are sexually least active during hot seasons. High environmental temperature upsets the normal physiological functions affecting spermatogenesis in males and ovarian activity in the females. 82% of services take place in November. Even under A.I. conditions, 65% of the inseminations of the year are being carried out during the months of September to February. Thus 80% of buffalo calvings are recorded only in the months of July to December and minimum in hotter months. With judicious management practices such as heat detection, protection from thermal stress, adequate and balanced ration and optimum time of insemination, the calvings in buffaloes could be evenly spread round the year to a great extent.

Silent Heat

Silent heat refers to normal follicular development and ovulations without the behavioural signs of estrus.

In summer the extreme climatic stress coupled with increased day light reduces the incidences of buffaloes coming in regular heat. During this time other reproductive problems like repeat breeding and pregnancy losses are also increased. It is generally felt that most of the buffaloes do have sub-functional ovaries causing weak or silent oestrus (in 60% cases) and such incidences are even higher than the true anestrous, especially in summer.

The research workers are trying to find out the causes of these disorders of ovarian origin and are successfully trying to correlate them with the lack of management, nutritional status of the animal and hormonal (serum gonadotrophins and steroids) profiles.

However, if due to excessive environmental stress the CL in buffaloes does not regress or partially regresses (in non-pregnant condition), it will continue to secréte progesterone and will inhibit further release of LH, thus the buffaloes will go in a state of anestrus or subestrus conditions, so long as CL does not completely regress.

Corrective Measures

For animals which either do not manifest oestrus or are in a state of silent oestrus or sub-oestrus firstly need managemental attention rather than therapies.

Two or three examinations with an interval of a week between each, will reveal that most of them are cases of apparent anestrus. In such cases simple utero-ovarian massage and close detection of oestrus will elleviate these conditions in most of the cases.

In extreme summer condition these animals should be protected from direct solar radiation by maintaining them in shaded half walled sheds. If possible animals be given showers in addition to wallowing facilities particularly at mid-day during April, May and June.

Parading vasectomized bulls for heat detection can be gainfully employed at organised/large farms. Since in summer buffalo bulls soon lose libido, replacement by young high libido bulls may be thought of where it is applicable.

Painting of Lugol's Iodine

The external is swabbed thoroughly with Lugol's solution (B. Vet. Co, Iodum 5 g, pot, iodíde 10 g, distilled water 100 ml) with the help of a metallic swab holder (46 cm.) and vaginal speculum- double application of this solution is sometimes recommended at week's interval. It is presumed that application of Lugol's Iodine on the cervix causes local irritation and bring about reflex stimulation of anterior pituitary for secretion of gonadotrophins and thus cyclicity starts.

Some workers have used estrogen and progesterone in anaestrus and sub estrus cows with encouraging success. The idea behind using small doses of these hormones are to act as a positive fed back at the hypothalamus level to release gonadotrophin releasing hormone (Gn-RH) and simultaneously sensitize the gonadotrophas in the anterior pituitary so that Gn-RH may act fully to stimulate more release of gonadotrophins.

It should be noted that the method can never be considered as a substitute for good management since use of hormonal therapy might also lead to inherent weakness in the progenies.

Use of prostaglandin ($PGF_2\alpha$) induces luteolysis resulting in sharp fall of serum progesterone level and thus helps to bring back normal oestrus cycle. Like hormonal therapy, prostaglandin therapy also can not be recommended as a substitute of good management.

Repeat Breeding

A repeat breeding in cow or buffalo is the one which has normal oestrus, oestrus cycles as well as reproductive tract and has been bred three or more times by a fertile bull or semen yet failed to conceive.

It is possible that pathology which cannot be detected by normal clinical methods may be present which include among others, failure of fertilization, an ovulation and delayed ovulation, tubal obstructions, early or latent embryonic mortalities, poor breeding and management techniques including genetic, nutritional and infectious factors. Endometritis in many cases has been found to play major factor for causing repeat-breeding. Endometritis is caused by sporadic uterine infections by a varieties of microorganisms such as *C. pyogenes*. *Coliforms*, *Pseudomonas aeruginosa*, *Streptococci* etc., viral and fungal agents along with mycoplasmal agents may also cause endometritis in cattle and buffaloes. The condition follows mainly parturition, especially abnormal ones; abortion dystokia, retained placenta, genital prolapse, uterine inertia, traumatic lesions in the uterus, cervix and vagina. Endometritis may also occur in cows and buffaloes after coilus or after AI under unhygienic conditions.

Appropriate antibiotic treatment is advocated after conducting antibiotic sensitivity tests where repeat breeding is associated with infection of the tubular genitalia.

Daily examination of repeaters is necessary to correct the conditions arising from ovarian dysfunction. Anovular heats can be detected from the absence of palpable C.L. during dioestrus. Intramascular injection of 25 mg of progesterone during early heat may help inducing ovulation.

The golden rule, prevention is better than cure applies more appropriately to reproductive problems. The incidence can be kept under control by adopting methods such as: (1) improved feeding and management, (2) providing hygienic surroundings at the time of calving, (3) asceptic precautions at the time of inseminations, and (4) educating farmers on detection of heat and maintenance of breeding records.

Weaning

Separating calf from its mother at a very early age is a bit difficult in buffaloes due to high motherly instinct. Since the method is important to assess dam's milk production and to feed calf according to live weight a substitution technique could be followed.

A single calf is substituted for let-down of milks in a number of buffaloes and the real calves are weaned just after birth. It can be achieved by putting blinkers (materials used to shut off the side views of buffaloes) during parturition and subsequently soiliing the body of substituted calf with placental secretions. The dam starts licking the substituted calf after removal of blinkers.

Calf Mortality

Buffalo calf mortality rate under one month of age averages about 10% and varies from 3-30% in individual herds. Losses upto 50% have occurred in large dairy herds. A calf mortality rate of 20% can reduce net profit by 38%.

A number of factors considered responsible for this hazard, are discussed below:

Antibodies are not transferable from buffalo dam to her fetus through placental membranes and thus they are susceptible to various virulent diseases. In buffalo calves inspite of feeding colostrum, a low antibody titre exists. Immunoglobulin levels have been reported to be 29.73 mg/ml it day olds and the quantity increase to 35.66 mg/ml on the second day of life. On the other hand in one estimate it has been noted that colostrum which is the only source of immunoglobulin for the buffalo calf, contains 68.75 mg of immuglobulin per ml on the first day, 23.75 mg/ml on the second day and 1.01 mg/ml on the fifth day of lactation.

Certain meteorological influences may have an effect on calf mortality rate. During the winter months, mortality may be associated with the effects of cold, wet and windy weather while during the summer it may be the hot, dry weather.

Most of the deaths occur during autumn and winter months before the age of 3 months. The causes of mortality in order of priority have been found (i) Pneumonia, (ii) Enteritis, (iii) Toxaemia/Septicemia, (iv) Worm infestation, (v) Bloat etc.

The cause of high mortality in male calves could also be due to neglecting tendency by the management particularly regarding feeding.

Some of the prescribed managemental practices including feeding practices may be followed for minimizing the mortality rate.

Housing

In commercial herds, calves after weaning may be kept in groups in large pens where individual feeding is advocated. In small herds calves after weaning should be kept in separate pens (24 sq. ft.) upto 3 months of age to avoid suckling instinct. The methods will eliminate the possible calf scour and parasitic infestation.

Feeding Colostrum

It is the milk secreted by the udder immediately after parturition and for the following 3-5 days. It contains 20% or more protein a little more fat, 10 to 100 times more vitamin A. three times more of vitamin D and may be tinged pink due to blood corpuscles. It acts as a natural purgative for the calf, cleaning from its intestines the accumulated faecal matter (meconium). Of much greater importance, it is through the medium of the colostrum, antibodies which protects against various bacteria and viruses are supplied to the new born calves. Colostrum coagulates at about 80^0 to 85^0 C and can not therefore be boiled.

The calves at birth after weaning should be fed colostrum within 2 hrs. and its feeding should continue for a period of five days at the rate of 1 to 1.5 kg per day.

In case the dam does not give colostrum a substitute of equal nutritive value prepared from 2 eggs and an ounce of castor oil may be fed for builiding up resistance. It may be necessary to inject dam's serum to such a calf for augmenting antibody titre in the body. The feed efficiency ratio of buffalo calves is as high as 1 kg. gain per 1.16 kg. dry matter. Milk feeding schedule is given in tabular form. It is necessary to provide milk to weaned calves at body temperature preferably with supplements to make up the deficiencies of Fe, Cu, Mg, Zn and Mn. Green fodder containing upto 100 gram dry matter may be offered daily from 15 days of age onwards so that it stimulates early rumen development.

Table 5.3. Milk feeding schedule

Age (days)	*Colostrum (kg.)*	*Body weight (kg.)*	*Milk (liters)*
1–5	1 to 1.5	—	—
6–15		Upto 25 kg.	1.0
11–15		26–30	2.0
15 and above		31–40	2.5
		41–45	3.0
		46–50	3.5
		51–55	4.0
		56–60	4.5
		60 and above	5.0

Feeding Antibiotics

Antibiotics are necessary in calves below 3 months of age to overcome certain stress conditions developed due to clinical or sub-clinical type of scour. These drugs are usually unnecessary in calves above 3 months as by this time rumen starts functioning and antibiotics are liable to interfere in normal functioning of ruminal microbes.

Feeding Milk Replacer

The objectives of feeding milk replace to calves are primarily to reduce the cost of raising buffalo calves and also to save milk for human consumption. Milk replaced may be fed as detailed in Tabular form. It may be noted that there is a gradual decrease in milk and corresponding increase in milk replaced at the rate of 200 g milk substitute per kg milk reduction. The general principle to be followed for calculation of milk requirement is that *it should be half kg. less than one tenth of the body weight*. It is also necessary to give a minimum of 1 litre of milk per day with milk replaced and the mixture should be diluted about six times with warm water to provide a drink in suspension form.

DISEASE

The most prevalent diseases of buffaloes are much the same as those of cattle, viz. rinderpest, foot-and-mouth disease, haemorrhagic speticaemia and anthrax. Buffaloes are generally less susceptible than cattle to foot-and-mouth disease but, when contracted, its debilitating effect may be disastrous: an attack during growth may cripple the animal for life, and if it occurs soon after calving often the entire lactation is affected. Buffaloes are much less susceptible than cattle to rinderpest, when managed under comparable conditions; the Egyptian buffalo is reported to be immune to natural infection. They are often infects with trypanosomes but the disease runs a chronic course giving rise to no visible symptoms. They are also infested with most of the larger parasites of cattle but the extent of the damage caused is often less noticeable. As would be expected, the incidence of liver-fluke is higher than in cattle. Of the arthropod parasites, the stable fly (*Stomoxys calcitrans*) and the so-called buffalo fly (*Siphona exigua*) attack buffalo more than cattle. On the other hand buffaloes are less affected by ticks but, as calves, they may be sorely tried by lice and mange mites.

6

Reproductive Technology in Cattle

Whether practitioner in the field, research worker in the laboratory, or educator of the next generation of veterinarians, delegates to this Congress are more or less bound to be confronted with questions – both technical and ethical – about how the "*new reproductive technologies*" (NRTs) are advancing cattle breeding, and how we veterinarians assess these developments. In this paper our aim to briefly answer the first question and offer some personal views on the second.

It is safe to say that virtually all people entering the veterinary profession do so as a result of their interest in animals. Later, that interest may become modified into a preoccupation with other organisms or factors affecting animals – parasites, microorganisms and disease processes for example – but the whole animal remains a principal focus of their work. The same used to be true of those of us who chose to specialize in reproduction. The fact that, uniquely, our discipline leads us to see the whole animal as only one component of the reproductive cycle.

The advent of in-vitro manipulation of gametes has shifted the emphasis of the NRTs from the diploid to the haploid half of the cycle, and this, we think, can affect the perspective of scientists who use them; the temptation is to share Samuel Butler's view that "A chicken is only an egg's way of making another egg". In my opinion there are dangers in adopting such a narrow viewpoint – dangers that veterinarians are in a privileged position to avoid.

Artificial Insemination

The oldest, the most widely used and the most beneficial of all the NRTs, AI is still developing. There are abundant reviews of how AI, in conjunction with intense selection and progeny testing, has had such an enormous effect on improving dairy production and how the advents of "*fixed time*" AI, and of sperm "*sexing*" (the separation of X- and Y-bearing sperm) are beginning to extend its usefulness even further. It has even been speculated that the major route of transgenes into the cattle population is likely to be, not through transgenic embryos as might be thought, but through transgenic spermatogonia transplanted into the testes of disseminating bulls by refinements of techniques pioneered in the laboratory of Brinster and his colleagues. Sometimes forgotten is the crucial role played by AI in all but eliminating so many venereal diseases in cattle – a role facilitated by the ability to hold frozen semen pending health checks on bulls. Thus, the reintroduction of the use of fresh semen in the interests of maximizing the number of AI doses per ejaculate is not without risk. Improving sperm cryopreservation so that the yield of straws per ejaculate is not reduced by freezing could eliminate any such risk.

A concerning corollary of the increase in milk production that has been brought about through AI is the concomitant decline in fertility. Manifestations of this confront veterinary practitioners every day and it is they who can bring signs of infertility to the fore. More or less elaborate schemes to counteract the problem, including the use of various NRTs, have been proposed but, in the long run, it may be more profitable to seek remedy through a fuller understanding of the causes of the decline, which can only come from research.

Embryo Transfer

In my opinion, the development and application of *embryo transfer* (ET) in cattle has been an excellent example of how the veterinary profession should interact with sister organizations for the good of animal production. The collegiality of veterinarians, animal scientists and biologists in the International Embryo Transfer Society (IETS) is exemplary and has paid important dividends, notably in the elaboration of internationally accepted procedures for moving embryos around the world. The history and current status of ET have been reviewed recently, describing how it has evolved through "*three generations*" – the first with embryos derived from donors (*in vivo*), the second with embryos produce in vitro, and the third including further in-vitro techniques, notably somatic cell nuclear transfer and transgenesis.

More than half a million (538,312) bovine embryos were reported to have been transferred in 2002, more than half of them (52%) after on-farm freezing and thawing and 15% of them having been produced in vitro. North America is still the centre of most activity (35% of the transfers) but this is static or declining in contrast to South America where ET is expanding and accounted for 22% of the world's transfers in 2002. Europe and Asia each reported about 17% of the total number of transfers in 2002. There is general agreement that a severe limitation to the more widespread use of ET is the problem of reliably inducing superovulation in selected donors, as will be discussed elsewhere in this Congress. Transvaginal ultrasonically guided "*Ovum Pick Up*" (OPU) at frequent intervals, in combination with *in-vitro fertilization* (IVF), is proving a more efficient route to producing embryos from individual donors where facilities and skills permit. Embryo sexing is quite widely practised; in Canada in 2002, almost 3800 sexed embryos were transferred, one-third of them after freezing and thawing.

ET is the NRT that has most directly involved large animal veterinary practitioners. However, their participation in routine field ET, which was absolutely essential when ET first became commercial in the early 1970s and collection and transfer were performed surgically, has gradually devolved, much as AI did earlier. In North American ET practices at least, it is suggested that the devolvement will continue. This is perhaps understandable, given that the challenge of putting a new technique to practical use has long since passed, but it is important to note that the need for veterinary involvement remains. Certification procedures demand it, for one thing, but, much more importantly, so do the proper appreciation of the potential of ET in disease control and investigation. A particularly good example of the importance of such an appreciation is the demonstration of how a non-cytopathic strain of BVD virus can adversely affect the production and manipulation of bovine embryos in vitro – essential components of the most recent NRTs discussed below. However, before embarking on that discussion, let us just remember that the proper transfer of embryos (however skillfully they may have been manipulated in vitro) to properly selected recipients, is an inescapable component of most animal biotechnologies and deserves corresponding veterinary attention.

Production of Embryos In Vitro

Bovine embryo production in vitro (IVP) is now a well-established and reasonably efficient procedure. It has proved its worth in improving the yield of embryos from designated donors subjected to OPU, salvaging irreplaceable genetics following slaughter in the face of infectious disease control or in culling for other reasons, and producing virtually all the thousands of embryos currently used for scientific research, including efforts to produce embryonic stem cells. The constituent oocyte maturation (IVM) and embryo culture (IVC) techniques are integral parts of the procedures for cloning by somatic cell nuclear transfer (NT) and facilitating the production of transgenic cattle that produce valuable pharmaceutical proteins in their milk. IVF by intracytoplasmic sperm injection (ICSI), so prominent in human assisted reproduction, is feasible in cattle, even with freeze-dried sperm, but is not yet widely applied. The fact that IVF embryos cultured in the sheep oviduct survive cryopreservation as well as do embryos collected in vivo indicates that it will eventually be possible to achieve similar survival of all frozen IVP embryos. Rather that try to review this immense field even briefly, let us consider four generalities that have emerged from the work and which are, we think, of special veterinary relevance.

The first generality is that the failures that have accompanied the development of IVP are proving every bit as instructive as the successes. Early embryonic loss and the "*Large Offspring Syndrome*" for example, have plagued IVP and cloning even though they can be largely avoided with appropriate culture systems. However, they have also been invaluable in focusing attention on the epigenetic effects of the environment from the earliest stages of development. This, in turn, has made us aware that "*insults*" to an early embryo - even inadequate maternal nutrition in vivo - can have effects that become manifest very much later. Clinicians responsible for the care of recipients carrying fetuses derived from manipulated embryos, especially clones, therefore need to be prepared to encounter losses much later in pregnancy than they normally do. Investigation of these syndromes is bringing together studies of embryology, gene regulation, "*hallmark pathologies*", physiology, and perinatology - a combination that is surely tailor-made for veterinary scientists of many stripes.

The second generality is that research makes us rethink some established dogmas in reproduction. Thus, early notions that "*genotype is everything*" (and the recipient relatively unimportant), which have underpinned the application of ET, clearly need to be tempered as our knowledge of epigenetics extends. Such extension may have both positive and negative effects. On the one hand, identification of "*intrinsically superior recipients*" for transferred embryos should eventually bring benefits to all aspects of bovine reproduction. On the other, the "identical" phenotypes anticipated to result from cloning may exhibit more variation than expected and desired.

Third in the list of generalities is the truism that initially complex techniques become simplified as they are put to use in the field, often in veterinary practice. ET itself, embryo manipulation and cryopreservation are examples and cloning may follow. The simpler the technique, the wider its applicability, making the prospects for NRTs benefiting animal production in less advanced countries a little brighter.

Our final generality is that a veterinary education is second to none as a starting point for those keen to take the NRTs to the next stage of newness, whatever that may be. For a research career, that education will have to be extended of course, but whether the choice is to explore the wonders of the haploid or diploid generation, a broad appreciation of the indivisibility of the two is a decided advantage. Practitioners, enjoying respect for their knowledge of animals and their welfare, will play an increasingly important role in influencing public perception of the NRTs, potentially a major impediment to their use. As a profession and as teachers, we should feel obliged to make good use of our privileged position both directly and through the students we educate.

Reproduction

Much of commercial animal production depends upon reproduction processes, for example, egg-laying in poultry, milk production in cows, sheep and goats. Selection for the development of these economically important traits has been undertaken over a comparatively long time. The speed with which improvement can be made or selection pressure applied has been improved by modern animal breeding techniques, amongst which is artificial insemination, record keeping on the farm, the use of computers and ease of communication.

Like any other character on which improvement is concentrated over many generations, there is the likelihood of a plateau being attained. So far, increases in two important characters associated with reproduction in the dairy cow and hen are still occurring.

It has been established that characters associated with reproduction have a low heritability. Most estimates place the heritabilities of milk production in cattle at 0.3 and of egg production in fowls at between 0.3 and 0.4. Too much must not be made of heritability estimates because their accuracy is directly related to the number of records examined and has only complete validity for those animals at that time.

If reproductive processes cannot be easily improved by the technique of selection, it emphasizes the importance of understanding the physiological processes involved. This permits us to devise routines of careful husbandry and, with the employment of the full resources of preventive medicine, to make sure that the genetic potential is fully realized.

Comparative Physiology of Reproductive Processes

The domestic and companion animals embrace two of the main divisions into which higher forms of life are divided, mammals and birds, each having different reproductive systems. In mammals, from the smallest per mouse to the elephant, the developing embryo remains within the uterus of the female until it has reached a relatively advanced stage of development, when it is able to walk or crawl round to the udder of its dam and suckle. The hen, after a successful mating, lays a fertilized egg that has to be incubated, that is, kept at a suitable temperature and humidity, and regularly turned. When the developing embryo, the chick, has reached a sufficiently advanced stage of development, it pecks its way out of the egg-shell to begin its independent existence.

MALE

Testes

The genetic material of the male of every species, that is to say the genes being contributed to the next generation, are carried in the spermatozoa or sperms, produced in large numbers in the two testes which in all mammals are of equal size. In birds, only the right testis is functional. In order that there may be the same number of chromosomes in the new individual that begins its life after the sperm has penetrated the ovum, there is a process of halving of the number of chromosomes of the developing sex cells of both male and female.

There are minor variations in the anatomy of the male reproductive organs of the various species.

Position of the testes

The two testes are held in the scrotum, the small skin-covered sac between the thighs of most animals. The boar and the tom-cat have the scrotum placed posterior below the anus. Some have the testes lying horizontally in the scrotum (stallion), most lie vertically; but all are outside the body. This is because the production of spermatozoa and their storage can only proceed normally at a temperature of several degrees below that of the body. One can notice

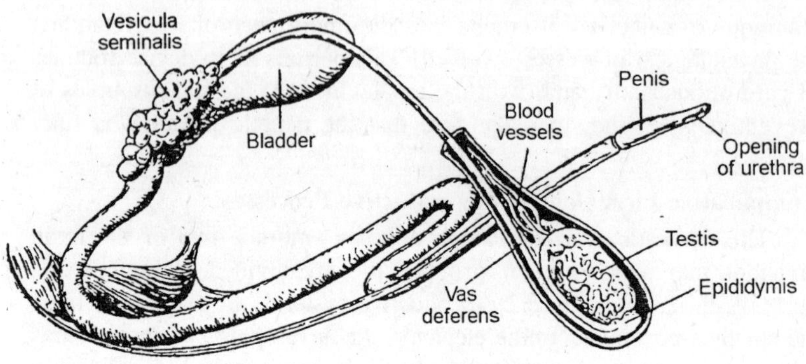

Fig. 6.1. Reproductive organs of the bull.

that during hot weather, the muscles holding the scrotum relax so that the testes are held at a lower level. During very cold weather, it has been found that the internal scrotal temperature is between 3 and 5°C less than the body temperature.

Rig or cryptorchid

Occasionally one or both testes do not get drawn into the scrotum during development before birth and, since the opening into the abdomen becomes narrower (the inguinal ring) after birth, the animal has reduced fertility. The defect in the animal causes it to be known as a cryptorchid or rig. If there is bilateral cryptorchidism, the animal is likely to be sterile because the temperature within the abdomen prevents the formation of sperms. This is thought to be an inherited defect, so that any animal showing it should not be used for breeding. It is a defect that appears more frequently in horses and pigs than in ruminants. When an animal reaches the age of puberty, the process of producing the sperms takes place in the substance of the testis from special cells, the spermatagonia, lining the closely packed seminiferous tubules. From here they pass into the long coiled tube of the epididymus (in the bull, this can be up to about 150 m in length). Entering at the top, or head of the epididymus, the sperms steadily get moved along by the contractions of its thin muscular walls and the action of its own movement, thus gradually progressing through the central section, closely attached to the testis, and along the protruding tail at the other end. From here they enter the larger tube, the vas deferens, and ascend the spermatic cord into the abdomen; finally they enter the urethra, from which they may be ejaculated from the penis.

The sperm reach maturity as they travel along the epididymus. Within the abdomen are situated the accessory sex organs, the seminal vesicles, prostate and Cowper or bulbo-urethral glands. They discharge their contents into the urethra, the tube that carries the sperms to the exterior.. These glands vary in size and activity with different species, e.g. in the boar the bulbo-urethral glands are large, but are absent in the dog. In the fluid of their secretions are salts, buffer and sugar to activate and nourish the rapidly moving sperms, as well as providing additional fluidity.

Each sperm consists of a head, in which is contained the chromosomes within a relatively large nucleus, covered by the acrosome, or cap. The small-mid-piece ends in the long tail, whose lashings help to propel it forwards.

The vas deferens enters the urethra at the spot where this tube comes from the neck of the urinary bladder. It is here that the secretions of the accessory sex organs mix with the sperm to produce the semen.

Penis

This is the copulatory organ and has important modifications in shape. In all animals it lies within the protection of the sheath, attached to the underside of the abdomen. This is lined with a membrane in which there are secretory glands, and which is continuous over the penis itself. That of the stallion has an enlarged end, with the whole organ provided with a plentiful blood supply. When sexually aroused, the blood supply is greatly increased, causing enlargement and protrusion from the sheath. In ruminants, there is an 'S' bend or sigmoid flexure which straightens during mating to permit the penis to emerge from the sheath. The ram and the goat have a thin urethral process at the tip of the penis.

At joining with the ewe, this rotates within her vagina, but is coiled in the billy-goat. The boar's penis has a twisted or corkscrew glans at its end; while in the dog there is a thin bone towards the tip, grooved underneath to take the urethra. It also has an enlargement behind it that swells during copulation, tightly gripping the interior surface of the bitch's vagina. The tom-cat has small projections pointing backwards.

Male mating behaviour

All the male farm and companion animals show characteristic behaviour at mating, that is to say, when they are brought into contact with a receptive female. To be willing to receive the male, she must be at a particular stage of her oestrous cycle during which she will show various signs of 'heat' or oestrus.

With the horse, a species in which hand or controlled mating is the common system, the mare thought to be in oestrus is brought into the presence of the stallion. If this procedure is attempted when the mare is not on heat, the mare may violently repulse him. Thus, when the mare is brought to the stallion, spoken of as a 'teasing', it is important to have solid fences or a gate between them. Should the mare be receptive, she will stand quietly and mating can safely follow.

The stallion and the bull show characteristic upward turning of the head, curving of the upper lip and flaring of the nostrils, spoken of as the 'flehmen'. Particular odours are associated with the different sexes, known as pheromones. Those produced by the female in oestrus help in her identification by the male; those produced by the male help to provoke receptivity in the female. With sheep and with pigs and cattle under some systems of management, where mating is uncontrolled, the identifying pheromones play an important part in the mating process.

Disorders of Reproduction in the Male

There can be a number of reasons for a male animal being incapable of producing normal semen, or there may be disease or injury involving the external genitalia that may interfere with his capacity or willingness to mate.

Testes

Injury may cause inflammation and swelling of one or both testes, a condition known as orchitis. An infection of the skin of the scrotum can also affect fertility. Any general infection that causes a raised temperature will inevitably cause a temporary sterility. There may be infection of either or both testes from blood-borne organisms, and routine examination by palpation should be made before purchasing any male animal or before the beginning of a mating season.

Epididymitis

Infection and enlargement of the epididymus, particularly in the ram, is by no means uncommon. In Australia, New Zealand and parts of Latin America, infection with *Brucella ovis* has been a problem, although several other species of bacteria can also cause inflammation in the epididymus. There is initial swelling, most marked in the protruding 'tail', easily felt at the lower end of the testis. It is a wise precaution to make a manual examination of a bull's testes before using him. Carefully and gently done, it can detect changes in the organ itself and in the associated epididymus. The normal gland feels smooth and uniformly tense but not hard.

Method of Examination

If a ram is being examined, he should be up-ended and held, sitting on his rump, by an assistant. The testes should be gently taken to lie in the palms of the hands, and the substance of each is felt to locate any area of inflammation, causing increased tenseness. A hardness will be felt if there has been fibrous tissue laid down after infection. The thumb and forefinger can then proceed to feel the epididymus, starting at the head and going down to the tail, before going upwards to the vas deferens part of the spermatic cord. There should be no thickening here or break as it mounts towards the inguinal ring, through which it passes into the abdomen.

The sheath, lined with the prepuce, can become infected, which may follow partial blockage of the urethra from calculi or small stones formed in the urine. The inflammation caused by this state of affairs has been called a balanoposthitis. It is a condition more commonly seen in wethers than in rams, goats or bulls. It demands veterinary treatment without delay. Bulls may be affected by a somewhat similar condition in which the prepuce prolapses, that is, it becomes slack, not being held in place by the muscles that normally do so. The tip of the penis is frequently seen protruding from the everted prepuce. Amongst bulls, it is often those of the beef breed that show this disorder when out at pasture, being especially common in zebu breeds, whose sheaths are always more pendulous. The treatment consists of clipping away the long hairs around the sheath and then carefully washing the part in warm, soapy water. Using more warm water, gently massage the tissues to increase the circulation. After drying, place some mild disinfectant ointment on the part. After repeating this procedure several times, it should become possible entirely to replace the everted tissue and return the penis to its normal position in the sheath.

More rarely, there may be injury to the penis, or inability to withdraw the penis from the sheath because of adhesions. Rest alone may bring about recovery, otherwise investigation under anaesthesia becomes necessary.

Occasionally, a male animal of reproductive age will show an unwillingness to mate with receptive females. This failure of libido can have several causes, apart from the effects of systemic or localized infection. Young rams need to be mixed with older fertile rams to encourage sexual activity. Beef bulls are often slow to begin service after reaching puberty at about 10 months and lose sex drive before dairy bulls, at about 6 years.

Bulls that have been successfully used in artificial insemination centres may suddenly refuse to serve or there may be failure of erection. This may be due to some accidental painful experience during service, but often the cause is difficult to ascertain. The use of a new 'teaser' cow of different appearance, or by simply resting the bull for a month or two may restore sexual vigour.

It is perhaps not surprising that the sperm cell concentration falls and the proportion of sperm showing defects rises during the hottest months when bulls of the European breeds are used in tropical countries. One recent study in West Africa showed that with lower temperatures during the wet season, there was an improvement in sperm density and sperm morphology.

Artificial Insemination

The technique of collecting semen from particularly desirable male animals of the various breeds of farm and companion animals and transferring this to a receptive female of the same species, that is, inseminating her, is one that is widely used, particularly in the dairy industry. Improved methods of diluting and storing semen, especially of the bull, has made it possible to inseminate from 40,000 to 60,000 cows per year from a single bull. It has been pointed out that it would be possible for 100 superior bulls to inseminate all the cattle in the U.K.

Collection of Semen

There are three methods for collecting semen. The commonest is to use an artificial vagina, consisting of a double-walled cylinder into the interior of which the male thrusts his penis and the outer chamber, filled with water at blood heat simulates the female vagina. The ejaculated semen is collected in a glass tube at the opposite end. The artificial vagina is made of a hardened rubber outer cylinder and the interior consists of a thin rubber tube inverted over the outer case which has an opening into which warm water is poured to give an interior temperature of 45-55°C. The male is lead to a female in oestrus ('on heat') and as he mounts her, the penis is directed into the artificial vagina. At Artificial Insemination Centres for dairy and beef bulls, it is often not possible to have a cow in season (in oestrus) available. Well-trained bulls can be satisfactorily stimulated by the presence of a quite cow not on heat, and at many centres the use of a 'dummy' consisting of a stretched hide over a frame is used. This can permit collection without diversion of the bull's penis by the operator crouching inside the frame. Stallions normally need the stimulus of a mare in season.

The second method, used more often with the ram and goat but sometimes with old lame bulls, is to use an *electro-ejaculator*. Placed in the rectum, this passes an electric current through the accessory sex glands and, as the stimulation proceeds, semen is produced and collected.

The third method is not used as a routine measure but can be used if a sample of semen is required and a bull has not been trained to serve into an artificial vagina or no cow in oestrus is available. A gloved and lubricated hand is put into the rectum and the seminal vesicles are gently stroked against the pelvis. The ampullae are then massaged and the semen that begins to drip from the sheath is caught in a glass funnel fitted into a glass tube held under the sheath opening. If semen is to be collected from a stallion, a condom may be used.

The glass tube into which the semen is collected must be warm, close to body heat, to prevent cold shock. It must at once be placed in warm water to maintain this temperature unless the air temperature is high.

Evaluation of Semen

Before semen is used it is important to have an assessment of its quality. An approximate estimation can be made by rapid inspection of the whole ejaculate. It should appear uniformly milky with no extraneous material such as blood or pus. Routinely, at Artificial Insemination Centres, a sample is immediately taken and a sperm count made. The quantity of semen in an ejaculate and the density of sperms in relation to the accessory glandular secretions vary considerably from species to species and even within a species, individual animals may vary widely in their characteristic sperm density. The extent of this variation is seen from the generally accepted values.

Table 6.1. Characteristic sperm densities

Animal	*Volume ml/ejaculate*	*Sperm concentration million/ml*
Horse	60-100	100-150
Bull	0.5-12	1000-1800
Boar	200-300	200-500
Ram	0.8-1.2	2000-3000
Dog	3-25	4-540
Cock	0.5-2.0	800-6800

In normal semen, not only will the sperm count be within a stated range, but the sperm will show great activity and there will be no more than 10 per cent with any abnormality, e.g. lacking the acrosome or with broken, bent or incomplete tails.

Dilution of Semen

Normally, in all species, following checking on density and viability, semen is diluted by mixing it with diluting fluid the composition of which affords nourishment to the sperms, buffers the mixture to prevent accumulation of acid and contains antibiotics to counter bacterial action. The amount of dilution depends upon the species, but, as an illustration, bull semen that is to be kept in the deep frozen state is diluted 10 times with an egg-yolk citrate or skim-milk extender. This commonly takes place at 25°C, before cooling to 5°C, when an equal volume of diluent containing glycerol is slowly added. Fresh bull semen has an approximate concentration of 1000 sperm per ml and it is accepted that an effective fertilizing dose is between 5 and 12.8 million. It means that one ejaculation from a bull is sufficient theoretically to inseminate 1000 cows.

Deep-frozen Bull Semen

For many years following the discovery of the protective effect of glycerol, semen from bulls used to be frozen at –79°C and, so long as there was no rise to –69°C, there was only slow deterioration in fertilizing ability. Now the use of liquid nitrogen allows semen to be kept at –196°C. The form in which the semen is stored and the manner of its use have also changed. From storing in small glass ampoules, the common methods at present are either to put the individual dose into a plastic 'straw', a thin tube of polyvinyl with 0.25-1 ml capacity, or by pellets, the method favoured in the U.S.A. These are formed by placing a drop containing 0.075-0.1 ml of diluted semen into holes in a block of solid CO_2, the pellet so formed representing one dose containing 12-30 million sperms. This is stored in liquid nitrogen wrapped in foil or in storage tubes.

Insemination

A successful insemination depends upon three factors, the recipient female, the skill of the inseminator and the quality of the semen.

Whatever the species of female animal that is to be inseminated, all tend to release a ripened egg from the follicle in the ovary (ovulation) towards the end of the period of oestrus or soon after its ending. This indicates the best time to inseminate.

Mares

Although not widely used, except within large horse studs, the steady increase in the number of light horses being bred all over the world for recreational purposes has stimulated research into making deep-frozen semen available. The difficulty has been in finding a satisfactory protective dilutent, since glycerol tends to depress fertilizing ability. Larger numbers of spermatozoa per insemination is used to compensate. It has also been found by workers in North America that there is a substantial improvement in the volume of ejaculate according to the season, with an increase of about 38 per cent from winter to spring, with a higher density of sperms. Fertility with frozen semen is mainly within the range 50-65 per cent.

With fresh semen, without dilution, and using 10-50 ml for each insemination (containing 1-2 billion sperms), four mares could be inseminated from one ejaculation. The mare is held in a crush and with the tail bandaged and the vulva washed. The sterile insemination catheter is guided into the dilated cervical canal by a gloved and lubricated hand inserted into the vagina. The fertility from using fresh semen is comparable to that from natural service.

Cows

The oestrous cycle of European breeds of cattle has an average length of 21 days, with greater variation being shown by zebu breeds as well as a shorter time during which signs of heat are shown. Ovulation takes place at about 12 hours after signs of oestrus have ceased, but maximum fertility results from insemination 6-24 hours before this.

Frozen semen is thawed just before being used and, by means of the appropriate instrument, the semen is inserted into the front part of the cervix (the short connection between the uterus and the vagina) or it is put just into the uterus. To do this, the inseminator places one hand into the rectum to hold the cervix and bring it slightly forward, thus to guide the sterile plastic pipette or the plastic 'straw' to the internal opening of the cervix. The dose of semen is injected by means of a syringe if the pellet form of semen is used, or by the plunger of the special applicator if a 'straw' is used, following the removal of the plugged end.

Assessment of fertility is by calculating the percentage of cows holding to first service (i.e. first insemination). If a cow does not return to oestrus during the following 60 days, it is likely that she has conceived. It was wise practice to have confirmation of the cow's pregnancy, either by means of a rectal examination by a veterinarian, or by ascertaining the level of progesterone in the milk. The Milk Marketing Board in the United Kingdom began to offer the latter service to dairy farmers when the technique of detecting the raised level following conception became reliable and could be automated.

Continuing shortage of dairy products in tropical countries has encouraged the use of frozen semen from high-producing progeny-tested bulls of European dairy cattle for improving yields by cross-breeding with zebu breeds where the standard of nutrition and general management of herds of tropical dairy cattle has been sufficiently improved to allow practical utilization of the higher genetic potential.

The use of performance tested beef bulls for artificial insemination has not been so popular, although such services are widely available. The main reason is that beef cattle are most commonly kept under extensive systems of husbandry, allowing calves to run with their dams over relatively large areas. Thus there are difficulties in detecting cows in oestrus and arranging to have semen brought at the right time. An effective way of overcoming this difficulty is to use 'teaser' or vasectomized bulls which can have a 'chin-ball' attached to a head collar which will mark cows found by the teaser to be on heat. Another device is to use adhesive Kamar pads on the rumps of cows so that, when they come into oestrus and stand to be mounted by another cow, a clearly detected dye stains the hindquarters.

Sheep

Except in the Soviet Union and some eastern European countries, where problems of cost-effectiveness are not so closely considered and where there has been the need to rapidly improve production characters, the use of artificial insemination in sheep has not become widely used. For many years, freshly collected and diluted semen was used. The technique of deep freezing ram semen in pellet form is now available, but it is widely held that the intense selection pressure long exercised in Australia for superior wool quality, as well as the availability of rams of the meat-producing breeds, considered in relation to the comparative low value of individual ewes, makes an insemination service uneconomic.

The procedure of inseminating a ewe, found to be on heat by the use of a vasectomized ram wearing a marking harness, is to have her held in a crate or cradle that presents the hindquarters to the inseminator. The vagina is opened by a perspex cylinder, the interior illuminated and the pipette guided into the cervix.

Sows

Many European countries and part of the United States, where pig production is an important livestock industry, have identified superior boars through progeny testing and performance testing schemes. When an artificial insemination service is available, many small producers find it uneconomic to keep a boar, and large enterprises that are closed because of the imposition of strict disease control, use it to introduce new genetic material. The detection of oestrus in sows when no boar is present is by no means easy. There are certain indications, such as a degree of restlessness in the sow, some swelling and reddening of the vulva; but the best indication of true heat is the *standing test* when the sow stands still and permits an attendant to put his weight on her hindquarters. With gilts, however, up to one-third may not react to this test. It is more effective to allow such young females to be brought within the proximity of a boar when the smell of the pheromones from his salivary glands and the sounds he makes will provoke stronger signs of oestrus.

Because of the circular folding of the cervix in the sow, the rubber catheter used is also spiralled at its tip, thus locking into place. It has been the practice to make up an inseminating dose to a volume of 50 ml containing 2 billion sperms. This is slowly transferred over 8-10 minutes under gravity into the uterus.

At most centres where boar semen is collected, the use of an artificial vagina has been discarded in favour of the gloved hand method. Most boars, after training, will serve on a dummy sow. This consists of a padded metal frame with a canvas cover. The gloved hand of the collector firmly grasps the penis, with its ridges held between the fingers. The first part of the ejaculate, the accessary fluid, is not collected. In contrast to the swift ejaculation of the bull and stallion, it takes about 10 minutes to collect the sperm-rich and subsequent parts of the boar's ejaculate (100-350 ml).

FEMALE

The contribution made by the female to her offspring is two-fold. Firstly, she makes an equal genetic contribution as the male, passing half her genes in the ovum (egg), released at the end of the oestrous cycle from the ripened follicle on the surface of the ovary. Secondly, as a result of the environment that she provides within the uterus during the time of gestation of the developing offspring, many opportunities occur for things to go wrong; for example, nutritional deficiencies in the diet or infection by pathogens.

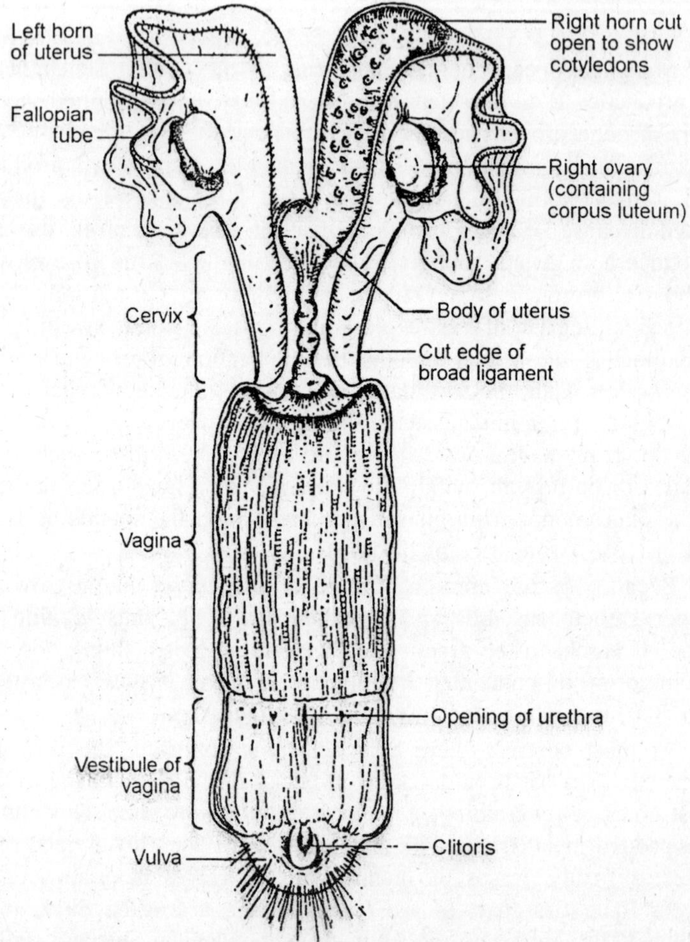

Fig. 6.2. Reproductive organs of the cow, slightly diagrammatic, seen from above.

Ovary

All farm and companion animals, except the fowl, have two ovaries located below the kidneys on both sides of the abdomen.

In the fowl, only the right ovary becomes functional. It is during the early cell divisions of the developing embryo within the uterus, that the first stage of meiosis occurs, but the second stage, which includes the actual formation of the ovum, only occurs as it reaches maturity during each oestral cycle. In the multi-ovular species, such as the pig, dog and cat, a number of eggs reach maturity and are released into the oviduct at the same time.

Oestrous Cycle

This is the term applied to the sequence of events that occur between the release of ova. Some species cycle throughout the year, others are seasonally polyoestrous.

The normal cycle can be divided into five parts. Just before oestrus there is a short pro-oestrous period when the ripening follicle in the ovary rapidly increases in size. The uterus enlarges and its serous lining thickens with its many glands becoming active. The lips of the vulva enlarge and, in ruminants, there is sometimes a slight discharge of clear mucus. In the bitch this discharge is blood stained.

Table 6.2. The oestrous cycle

Animal	*Length days*	*Time of year*
Mare	21 (19-26)	Spring and summer
Cow	21 (18-24)	Throughout year
Ewe	17 (14-20)	Autumn; Dorset horn and Merino and tropical breeds cycle throughout year
Goat	18 (18-21)	Autumn
Sow	21 (16-24)	Throughout year
Bitch	21 twice yearly	January-March; August-September
Cat	3-4 weeks	Spring; late summer; autumn

Table 6.3. Heat period and ovulation

Animal	*Duration of heat*	*Ovulation*
Mare	6 days	24 hours before the end of oestrus
Cow		
European	ca. 24 hours	14 hours after the end of oestrus
Tropical	3-7 hours	
Ewe		
British breeds	36 hours	Near the end of oestrus
Merino	48 hours	
Goat	24-48 hours	Near the end of oestrus
Saw	40-60 hours	30-40 hours after beginning of oestrus
Bitch	9 days	5-12 hours after the end of oestrus
Cat	3-6 days	26 hours after mating
	5-12 days if not mated	

During oestrus itself the vagina enlarges and the cervix relaxes. This is the time that the females of all species seek to mate with the male and will stand to do so. The time that this lasts varies, not only between species, but between breeds and individuals

When the period of heat ends it is succeeded by metoestrus, during which the ruptured follicle in the ovary fills with luteal tissue to form the corpus luteum, or yellow body. Dioestrus is the time that elapses before the beginning of the next oestrus. When an animal has a period of sexual rest she is said to be 'in anoestrus'. Now the ovaries are inactive and the uterus contracted. Sheep, goats, dogs and cats, especially in temperate regions, tend to have anoestrous periods lasting several months.

Pregnancy

The egg, after its release from the ovary, enters the fallopian tube through the distal expanded end and begins its descent towards one of the two horns of the uterus with which it connects. If there has been a normal mating, or the introduction of spermatozoa by artificial insemination, the upward swimming sperms very quickly reach the upper part of the fallopian tube. One sperm gains entry, although it is accepted that up to a million should be introduced when using artificial insemination. The first mitotic division immediately takes place. Further division occur in what is now known as the blastocyst as it enters the uterine horn and becomes attached to the lining membrane after several more days, the time taken varying from 12 days in the cow to 30 days in the mare.

As the embryo develops and a normal pregnancy proceeds, the developing embryo is enclosed within a thin-walled sac, the amnion, which itself is within and connected by the umbilical cord to another sac, the allantochorion. The latter becomes attached to the lining of the uterus. The form of this attachment varies with the species. In ruminants, there are a series of protuberances, the *cotyledons* or caruncles, about 120 in the cow and 80 in the ewe, arranged in four rows along each of the uterine horns. These provide the means for the dam's circulation to nourish the new offspring, now known as the foetus.

There is a different arrangement in the pregnant mare, sow, bitch and cat. These have a large number of small finger-like processes called *villi* making the connection between the allantochorion and the endometrium or lining of the wall of the uterus. In the mare and sow these are found all over the outer surfaces of the foetal sac, while in the bitch and cat it is only the central part that becomes vascularized (having a supply of blood from the mother). It is this foetal sac that is known in all mammals as the *placenta*.

Throughout its intra-uterine life, the foetus floats in the amniotic fluid which, in its turn, is surrounded by increasing amounts of allantoic fluid, together making up the foetal fluid. This may be as much as 20 litres at the end of the pregnancy in the cow.

Factors Controlling Fertility

It is a prime aim with farm livestock that young females should be fit to mate at as early an age as possible to permit the production of vigorous offspring of optimum size. A long life of regular breeding should follow such a rearing routine, assuming freedom from disease and a continuation of good husbandry. It requires careful attention to the feeding and management of the prospective dam from its birth.

Consider the growing female calf, the heifer, as an illustration of what should be done. There is a direct relationship between the level of nutrition given to a heifer calf and the age of puberty. Thus it is possible, by persistent high feeding from an early age, to obtain a successful mating when a calf is less than 15 months old. The first lactation yield of milk from such 'forced' females is almost always disappointingly low. Maximum lifetime production from cows is more likely to follow a rearing period, during which the female calf is fed a carefully balanced diet at a moderate level from weaning onwards and is mated for the first time at about 18 months of age.

With all the common domestic animals, the arrival of puberty comes before growth is complete. Fertility is likely to be low and uncertain, so the time of first mating is delayed to an extent that varies with the species.

Table 6.4. Age of puberty and mating

Animal	*Puberty*		*Mating*
	Mean, months	*Range, months*	
Mare	18	12-24	3 years
Cow	13	6-12	18 months
Ewe	10	6-12	18 months
Goat	7	5-9	18 months
Sow	7	6-8	8 months
Bitch	9	6-12	12 months
Cat	6	5-8	10 months
Rabbit	6	18	
Fowl	22 weeks	18-24 weeks	over 1 year

The filly foal will reach puberty at an age that is even further from the time that growth ceases, i.e. the age of maturity. It is therefore desirable to delay first mating until nearer that stage, if growth is to be uninterrupted and difficulties at parturition are to be avoided. With modern strains of crossbred ewe lambs, it has become increasingly common, on properties able to provide optimum nutrition during their first winter and good care at lambing, to undertake their mating at about 8 months. Fertility is below that obtained with mature ewes, but subsequent reproductive capacity does not appear to be adversely affected.

The endeavour with modern strains of gilts is similar. Many breeders may still be content with mating at slightly over 9 months at a weight of 130 kg, but it is the aim of progressive farmers to mate gilts two months earlier when their weight is likely to be close to 105 kg. A satisfactory breeding life and optimum litter size depends upon adequate feeding of a balanced diet, not only through each pregnancy, but during lactation and the dry period that follows.

Control of Oestrus by Hormones

A series of chemically identified and naturally produced hormones regulates the succession of events that have already been described as making up the oestrous cycle. They have three sources: from that part of the central nervous system called the hypothalamus, from the nearby anterior pituitary gland (both situated at the base of the brain), and from the ovary and uterus. It appears that with most species, there is an external stimulus necessary to initiate regular heat periods.

With small ruminants and the mare, it is the seasonal change in the day length that initiates the oestrous cycles after puberty, assuming normal temperature and optimum nutrition. With the mare, it is the increasing length of the daylight in the spring and, with the ewe, the decreasing daylight of autumn that has this effect.

The hypothalamus produces certain 'releasing factors' which act on cells in the nearby anterior pituitary gland to produce *follicle-stimulating hormone* and *luteinizing-hormone*. The action of the former is to stimulate the cells within the ovary to proceed to the ripening of the follicle, simultaneously bringing about a release of *oestrogen* into the circulation. Its main effect is to cause the various observable signs of heat.

It is immediately followed by production of luteinizing hormone, causing the cells in the ovary to secrete increasing amounts of *progesterone*. This is accompanied by the enlargement of the corpus luteum in place of the ruptured follicle. The effect of progesterone is to abolish all signs of oestrus, bringing about the state of anoestrus. If pregnancy follows, the level of progesterone in the circulation (and in the milk of a lactating cow) continues to rise until about the 20th day, but stays at a fairly high level until after the 40th day in this species. The placenta also produces progesterone as a function of maintaining pregnancy.

Apart from the central nervous control by the hypothalamus in producing successive releasing factors to the anterior pituitary, there is a powerful group of hormones, the prostaglandins, produced in various tissues; but one, prostaglandin $F_2\alpha$, from the uterus has the effect of causing the destruction of the corpus luteum, and thus the rapid diminution of circulating progesterone. In the non-pregnant animal this signifies the end of the dioestrous period of the normal oestrous cycle and the beginning of pro-oestrus. In the pregnant female it occurs when parturition or the birth process is coming close.

Detection of Pregnancy

It is desirable to be able to be sure that an animal is indeed pregnant at as early a time as possible. In some species, such as the mare, bitch and cat, where each individual is often under close observation, the missing of the succeeding heat period after mating is a hopeful indication of pregnancy. With herd animals, cows, sheep, goats and sows, such close observation may be difficult, although the keeping of records specifying the date on which mating began and the employment of marking techniques can provide information about the commencement of parturition.

Mare

Two methods of detecting pregnancy are commonly used. The most reliable is for a veterinarian to make a clinical examination. This may be done in one or both of the following two ways: a rectal examination is undertaken, during which the uterus is felt with the hand and arm inserted into the rectum. The best time for this to be undertaken is 35-40 days after mating. Sometimes an examination of the vagina is made using a speculum, for there are a series of changes in the lining cells, the amount of mucus present and the appearance of the external opening of the cervix.

The second method is to take a blood sample to see if there is present the special hormone produced in large quantities by the pregnant uterus. It is called 'pregnant mare serum gonadotrophin' and has both oestrogenic or follicle-stimulating and luteinizing properties. It is first demonstrable in the blood serum of the mare between days 38 and 42, reaches a maximum at about 60-65 days and disappears by the 150th day. A blood sample should therefore be taken between days 60 and

100. In the *mouse test* a small amount of the serum is injected twice daily for two days into each of four female mice 3-4 weeks old. When the mice are autopsied some 24 hours later, the test is positive if the uteri are some five times normal size.

In the *haemagglutinin inhibition test*, a sample of the mare's blood serum is diluted with acetone, and the resulting precipitate put into buffered saline to be incubated for one hour. Specially prepared sensitized sheep erythrocytes and anti-pregnant mare serum are mixed with increasing dilutions of the mare's serum. If the mare is pregnant, there will be no clumping together of the red blood cells.

This test has about a 90 per cent level of accuracy and is believed by some experts to be preferable to making repeated clinical examinations. These have become routine in many horse studs, but there is the possibility that the low levels of fertility commonly experienced amongst thoroughbreds in many countries may be in part due to this manual interference.

Cow

Until the mid-1970s, the most reliable method of ascertaining whether a cow previously mated, and not since seen to show oestrus, was already pregnant or barren was to have a clinical examination made per rectum. The various changes that take place in the size and position of the uterus of the pregnant cow can be most certainly detected when an examination is made after 90 days, but experienced veterinary practitioners can make accurate assessment a month or six weeks before this.

With the greatly increased accuracy that the use of a radio-immune assay for progesterone in the milk gives, especially when it was found possible to automate the procedure, it has become possible for organizations, such as the Milk Marketing Board of England and Wales, to offer their members a reliable diagnostic service. A sample of milk is taken from the cow between the 18th and 24th day following mating or artificial insemination and sent to the Milk Marketing Board laboratory. The result is sent back within a few days. Accuracy is over 90 per cent with negative results and a little over 80 per cent for positives.

Progressive dairy farmers, anxious to maintain high levels of production by endeavouring to have their cows produce a calf each year, use both aids to discover if mating or artificial insemination has been successful. A more recent development has been the discovery that some cows always have higher than normal progesterone levels.

These would account for the few false positive readings from the milk test, discovered later by the *per rectum* examination. A blood sample taken at the time of examination will detect such cows, for at this time progesterone levels are normally low.

Ewe and goat

A common and satisfactory way to monitor the occasion of the ewe being mated is to place a marking device on the ram. One widely used, first in Australia and New Zealand, but for many years by British sheep farmers, is the 'Sire-syn- harness. This has a socket in the harness that fits over the brisket, containing an easily changed block of raddle. If the colour is altered every 17 days, any ewe that does not conceive to a first service will have a second colour put upon her rump. For the valuable stud ewe, or nanny-goat, there are more sophisticated methods of pregnancy diagnosis available. These include using an ultrasonic foetal pulse detector. It has a probe that is moved over the bare or shaved surface of the abdomen immediately in front of the udder. Only when the pregnancy is over 60 days and after experience in its handling, is there likely to be an acceptable degree of accuracy. Beyond 70 days, radiography is very accurate but expensive.

Sow

Non-return to oestrus after 21 days and 42 days gives a clear indication that the sow is pregnant, but in large units where sows are often kept in stalls, signs of heat are often difficult to detect. There is available an ultrasonic foetal pulse detector in which a probe is placed on the abdomen or into the rectum. It works through the foetal pulse interfering with the transmitted signal. It is an expensive machine requiring a good deal of experience for effective use to be made of it.

There is also a method that requires the services of a laboratory. This involves the removal of a small piece of the lining of the vagina by a special instrument. A characteristic arrangement of the cells is shown by the pregnant sow, when the stained specimen is examined microscopically. The best time to test is between 18 and 25 days after mating.

Bitch and cat

Even if she is not mated, the bitch not infrequently has a false or pseudo-pregnancy. This state may persist for the whole of the 63 days that is the normal length of gestation, to end with the enlargement of the mammary glands and a behaviour pattern similar to the pregnant animal. A pregnant bitch tends to show behavioural changes, becoming quieter and more lethargic. There is a tendency to lay down subcutaneous fat and, if she is carrying many pups in utero, the abdomen will show distension by the 5th week. An infected uterus could be the cause of this, so it is better carefully to feel the uterus and the enlargements that are the growing foetuses. It is only easily done if she is not one of the large breeds and is of quiet disposition, so as not to resent this handling. It is most usefully done at about the fourth week of pregnancy. It should then be possible to feel the spherical swellings made by the foetuses along the horns of the uterus.

Because of the thinner adbominal wall in the cat, palpation is easier. If necessary, radiography can be used with a high degree of certainty after day 25 when ossification of bones has begun, and in skilled hands even earlier.

Parturition

The process of giving birth in mammals begins when the foetus has grown to a stage that permits it to fend for itself in the external environment. The procedure is controlled by a series of co-ordinated events, mediated through changing hormone levels in the circulation. These come from the central nervous system, the pituitary, the uterus, and from the corticosteroids produced in the adrenal glands of the dam and the foetus itself. It is important to be familiar with the normal length of the pregnancy, the gestation of each of the farm and domestic animals.

Table 6.5. Length of pregnancy

	Day	
Animal	*Mean*	*Average*
Mare	336	325-341
Cow: European	280	277-284
Zebu	286	284-288
Ewe	147	146-149
Goat	151	145-156
Sow	114	110-117
Camel	300	280-320
Buffalo	316	314-320
Bitch	63	60-66
Cat (queen)	63	60-66
Rabbit (doe)	31	30-33

A clear indication that birth is near is given by the enlargement of the mammary gland and teats of the dam. The lips of the vulva swell and may show some reddening, and there may be a slight haemorrhage. The ligaments attached to the sacrum relax in the cow, giving the hind quarters a sunken appearance.

The dam will almost always show behavioural changes as the period of gestation comes to an end. She will tend to go apart from the group and, if possible, seeks a quiet, secluded spot for giving birth.

When these premonitory signs occur, it is wise to bring the animals into special accommodation, a loose box for mares and cows which must be thoroughly clean and free from infection, well lighted and well ventilated, but without draughts. This accommodation should be in a quiet corner of the farm buildings, but of easy access to the animal attendant. It must have ample space without projections or encumbrances and thus should be larger than the usual stall or loose box. Plenty of clean bedding must be put down, a feeder at the right height from the ground, with drinking water always available. It is desirable for the parturient animal to have a day or two to become familiar with the place before the birth process starts. The nearness of parturition in the mare is shown by the enlargement of the mammary gland and a 'waxing' of the teats, sometimes with the escape of a few drops of colostrum. She may show patches of sweat by the elbows and flanks.

Normal Parturition

The effect of the changes in hormone secretion that occur when gestation comes to an end is to cause gradually increasing rhythmic contractions of the muscle fibres within the uterus. To begin with, in what is properly called the *first stage of labour*, these periods of contractions are not frequent and are interrupted by periods of rest. In the cow, these deep peristaltic waves that start at the distal end of the horn of the uterus and progress forward, occur every 15 minutes, become more frequent as the foetus is moved towards the cervix or vagina, until they occur every 2-3 minutes during the hour before the calf is born.

The cervix at the end of the vagina at this time becomes relaxed and enlarged to form a continuous canal, through which the foetus must pass, preceded by the allantochorionic sac.

It is at this stage that the foetus turns itself to be in the right position for being born. For the foal and puppy this means turning over with the head uppermost but, with the foal, calf and lamb, also an extension of the forelimbs. All foetuses at this stage extend their forelimbs forward, although many piglets are born with the hindlegs coming first. During this first stage, the dam is often restless, moving about or getting up and then lying down. It lasts from 3 to 6 hours, and by the time the second stage begins the dam lies to give birth.

The expulsion of the foetus or the second stage of labour is aided by contraction of the abdominal muscles in association with continuing uterine action. The allantochorionic sac breaks and much dark-coloured fluid comes from the vulva. As the head and shoulders of the foetus enters the cervical canal, a rise in oxytocin output from the posterior pituitary causes very strong muscular effort to force the foetus through to the outside, where it appears with the amnion or 'water-bag'. This is often broken by one of its feet or, with the mare, as it reaches the ground, or during the last part of its expulsion, and breathing starts. It is important to allow the umbilical cord connecting the newly born animal with the maternal membranes to break of its own accord following movement by the newly born animal or its dam as she gets up. This is important because blood-containing substances, that will give the young animal resistance to any pathogenic microorganisms in the surroundings, pass from the placenta at this moment.

This stage takes a varying time according to the species. It is shortest in the mare, where a mean time of 17 minutes is given and longest with the sow, who frequently takes over 4 hours before the last piglet is born. The last or third stage of labour is simply the expulsion of the foetal membranes or afterbirth. It is swiftest in the mare, for it follows the birth of the foal within about 1 hour, but with the cow it is about 6 hours. All the farm and domestic species, except the mare, normally eat their afterbirth.

The dam, except the sow, will shortly begin licking her offspring. Partly through this stimulation and that of hunger, the young creature will find its way to its dam's mammary gland and begin suckling. The importance of receiving *colostrum*, the first secretion of the mammary glands, lies in its high nutritive value and in its concentration of protective antibodies, the immunoglobulins. The capacity of the intestine to absorb these proteins diminishes rapidly after 36 hours, which emphasizes the need for anyone attending animals at this time to see that the newly born gets its share of colostrum as quickly as possible.

Ewes

The lambing ewe flock is, in the U.K., increasingly being brought inside to lamb. The winter housing of ewes has been found to be economically justified under certain conditions of soil and climate, but in most sheep-farming areas a more limited type of under-cover accommodation, for different groups of ewes as they come to lamb, achieves the object of reducing perinatal losses, that is losses amongst both ewes and lambs that occur just before, at the time of parturition or during the first few days after birth.

It is an important reason for adopting the practice of using marked rams at mating. This makes it possible to draft ewes into groups according to the time of lambing, so enabling the vitally important extra feed to be given during the last 6 weeks of pregnancy and then to bring them into sheltered surroundings for the actual lambing. Whether this is entirely indoors or in an area protected from the worst of the weather outside, it must be clean and quiet. If outside; adequate protection can be provided by straw bales formed into small lambing pens. So long as the nutrition of the ewe has been correct, and measures taken to prevent disease, there will be little difficulty and few losses.

Sow

It is the commonest practice to-day to put sows about to farrow in one of the many varieties of farrowing crate. In this multiparous species, with litters of 8-12 usually being born, loss of piglets from the sow lying on them was a problem that the farrowing crate has largely solved.

It is placed in a pen that should be 1.5-2 m wide. Typical measurements are 2.11 m (7 ft) in length by 0.76 m (2 ft 5 in) wide and 0.88 m (2 ft 10 in) high.

The sow enters through a door in the back of the crate and there must be a bar at the bottom attached to it, 228 mm (9 ins) from the floor and/or 228 mm (9 in) from the back of the door to prevent piglets being crushed by the rump of the sow as she lies down.

The crate permits the sow to get up and lie fully stretched out, but she is unable to turn around. Infra-red heating lamps are usually hung over the space away from the sow to attract the piglets from her side when not sucking. If the piggery is not well insulated or heated, it is advisable for the first few days at least to cover the area where the piglets run with hardboard to conserve heat. The concrete floor, if insulated, can be covered by sawdust or wood shavings, otherwise a covering of straw is warmer.

In the last part of pregnancy sows are very lethargic, but the mammary glands show much enlargement about 24 hours before farrowing begins. Now they show much restlessness and they will go through bed-making movements. By this time the individual teats and the mammary glands have enlarged and stand out. These periods of activity alternate with rest periods, but it is only about an hour before the first piglet appears that the sow will settle on her side and be still. The length of time that a sow takes in giving birth depends upon her age, fertility, breed and individual characteristics. Gilts, or maiden sows, take longer and often get up and turn over between the birth of the piglets. One large series of observations showed that as many as 45 per cent were born with the hind legs foremost. The sow expels most of her afterbirths along with the piglets, so that the second and third stages of parturition are more or less combined.

Most sows, when they have completed the process of giving birth, will stand and pass a lot of urine before lying again to suckle. It is at this moment that there is likelihood of overlying and crushing some of the last born piglets unless they have got themselves out of the way or been placed outside the farrowing crate by the attendant.

The bitch

The first stage of labour in the bitch reveals itself as increased restlessness; she will not eat, may pant and there is swelling of the mammary glands with milk already present. She will be in her nest for the second stage, the expulsion of the first foetus, which may take up to one hour. The bitch frequently pauses in her straining, once the water bag appears at the vagina, to lick it vigorously, so rupturing it. The head of the puppy then appears and the rest of its body is quickly expelled. Many puppies are normally born in the posterior presentation. There is much variation in the time taken by any particular bitch in giving birth to the rest of her litter. Some may rest for up to several hours between the first and second puppy, others give birth to their puppies at regular short intervals. The bitch expels the foetal membranes within 15 minutes of each birth and they are quickly eaten by her. The dark greenish uterine discharge which may be noted is normal.

Cat

The process is similar to that described for the bitch except that the number of kittens born is often less, rarely more than five. The time taken is less, with more regular time intervals and the uterine discharge is brown.

Care of the Newborn

Whatever the species, the good husbandman will do his best to see that the newborn creature finds its way to the mammary gland of its dam as speedily as possible after its birth in order that it may obtain the valuable colostrum, both for nourishment and to obtain the immunoglobulins that will help to protect it against some of the pathogenic microorganisms of its environment.

Disorders of Reproduction in the Female

Infection Following Parturition

It must be understood that there is a normal and varied bacterial flora in the vagina of all domestic animals. During and after parturition there is inevitable aspiration of some of these microorganisms back into the open cervix and the uterus. The normal defence mechanism against invading microorganisms comes into play and, in the vast majority of instances, within a comparatively short time, i.e. within days, the tract is free of infection.

If there has been difficulty over giving birth, i.e. dystokia, with damage to the epithelium lining the reproductive tract, then a more persistent and serious degree of infection may follow. In cattle particularly, this is likely to be associated with retention of the afterbirth, when a massive infection of the uterus inevitably occurs. The result of this state of affairs is that the dam cannot be mated again until the infection has been overcome and normal oestrous cycling has been established.

The method of treatment varies according to the severity of the case. It is often necessary to remove the retained afterbirth manually if there is a persistent uterine inertia that has not responded to treatment with such hormones as oxytocin and prostaglandin. Whenever, there is evidence of toxaemia in the dam, antibiotics are administered.

Occasionally, with the cow and mare, damage to the vagina and cervix may result in the persistent sucking-in of air, as well as the danger of recurring infection. An operation to repair the reproductive tract becomes necessary.

Another post-parturient abnormality which may occur following the third stage of labour in any species, but is commonest in ruminants, is prolapse or eversion of the uterus. Clearly, it is important to minimize the organ's contamination; so it should be wrapped in a clean towel until veterinary help arrives. In the cow, straining must be avoided during replacement, so a local anaesthetic is injected into the epidural canal at the first intercoccygeal space. After careful washing in warm, normal salt solution, the uterus will be carefully replaced by the veterinarian.

When this accident occurs in the ewe, it is not so difficult to replace the uterus if an assistant raises the hindquarters. If the afterbirth has not separated, the foetal cotyledons should not be forced away from the uterine caruncles, as they will be returned to allow normal separation later.

This is a very rare occurrence in the mare, although it appears likely to be a consequence if birth has to be by Caesarean section because of post-operative suture adhesions.

Infections During Pregnancy

Many infectious agents, bacteria, viruses, protozoa and fungi can prevent pregnancy or induce abortion. They can gain entry to the uterus and there produce a metritis, in two ways: (i) at the time of mating, or from infection introduced during artificial insemination; (ii) from the circulation, brought from a reservoir of infection (e.g. the udder) or from a general blood-borne pathogen.

Mare

There is often difficulty in obtaining a desired pregnancy in the mare, particularly in Thoroughbreds. Most commonly the reasons appear to be of a functional or physiological nature. Venereal infection is generally infrequent. With the exception of the specific venereal pathogen *Haemophilus equigenitalis*, the cause of contagious equine metritis, first introduced into the United Kingdom in 1977, and capsule types 1, 2 and 5 of *Klebsiella aerogenes*, the only other organisms implicated in endometritis in mares are species of streptococci or staphylococci that have managed to gain entrance to the uterus following foaling or as a result of 'windsucking' from defective closure of the lips of the vulva.

The venereal pathogens can gain entrance to the uterus through the stallion carrying infection at mating or from genital examination subsequent to service. To discover the nature of the infection and the appropriate treatment to be undertaken, a sterile swab is carefully introduced into the anterior cervix or uterus and bacteriological examination made. The sinus associated with the clitoris must be swabbed in checking for contagious equine metritis.

Abortion can be caused by infection by the virus, equine herpes virus I or rhinopneumonistis. This produces a mild infection of the lungs and respiratory tract which may not be noticed, but abortion mostly occurs during the last four months of pregnancy. Mares recover spontaneously and after 1-2 months will conceive.

In some countries, *Salmonella abortus equi* still occur although effective vaccines and drugs are available and can bring about its eradication. Again, the protozoon parasite, *Trypanosoma equiperdum*, causing dourine, is still found in some parts of the world. It is a serious and frequently fatal disease and all infected and in-contact animals should be slaughtered.

Cow

Bacteria

There are a number of venereal diseases of cattle, transmission being by the infected male. One of the commonest in both cattle and sheep is *Campylobacter vibrio foetus*, of which three different types are recognized, two found in cattle (*C. foetus venerealis* the most common, and *C. foetus* var. *intestinalis* type I) and the third (*C. foetus* var. *intestinalis* type II) sometimes in cattle but mainly in sheep, where it is not spread venereally. A bull can harbour the infection in his prepuce but show no symptoms.

During natural mating the infection is passed to the female and this is likely to prevent conception. If a new bull is used and there is a high proportion of cows and heifers returning to service, this is the infection that should be suspected. Tests can be made on a sample of vaginal mucus and washings from the bull's prepuce using a fluorescent antibody technique. Artificial insemination from a clean bull will permit pregnancy and most cows will overcome the infection and develop an immunity within a few months. Where artificial insemination cannot be used, such as in large beef herds or in developing countries, an effective vaccine is available and can be used to protect cows. Some reports indicate its use in curing bulls of infection.

The commonest cause of abortion in cattle in many countries has been infection with *Brucella abortus*. Brucellosis (Bang's Disease) causes undulant fever in man, although many other symptoms appear apart from a fluctuating high temperature. The cow's udder appears to be the reservoir of infection from one pregnancy to the next.

Infection is the result of grazing over infected pasture or from a cow licking the discharges from an animal that has aborted, or even the foetus itself. If a bull has the infection in his testes, it will have an orchitis and its semen is infective. When heifers or young cows are infected, there is a high incidence of abortions. Older cows that have been infected during earlier pregnancies may carry calves to full term, but these are often of small size and later suffer from scouring. This is a disease which can be passed to humans through the drinking of raw milk or by direct contact by those handling infected cattle. An effective attenuated live vaccine, S19, has been widely used. It must be injected into calves between 4 and 8 months old. When used conscientiously and consistently this will entirely prevent clinical disease, but does not eliminate the organism. With the greater accuracy of an improved complement fixation test and the use of a fluorescent antibody test, identification of infected cattle has become more certain. This has encouraged the establishment of abortion-free herds. Most temperate countries have, therefore, either already eradicated the disease or have embarked upon long-term eradication campaigns.

Mycoplasma infection (contagious granular vaginitis) is a widespread cause of infertility and occasionally of abortion. It may infect bulls. The organism is *Mycoplasma bovigenitalium* and can be transmitted by the bull, where it causes epididymitis. In cows it is also a cause of mastitis. It is often present in healthy cattle, causing pathogenic changes when resistance is lowered by other causes.

Viruses

Several viruses have been identified as the cause of infertility in cows. A common one appears to be identical with that known to cause infectious bovine rhinotracheitis which frequently appears as a nasal discharge, as well as infectious pustular vulvo-vaginitis (IBR-IPV virus). It is a venereal disease, causing a painful infection of penis and prepuce, making the bull reluctant to serve. When the vagina of a cow becomes infected following mating, the lips of the vulva show swelling and reddening within 24 hours, followed by red vesicles on the mucosa. There is much mucopurulent discharge and sometimes high temperature and lack of appetite. Recovery without treatment occurs within 2-3 weeks and abortion does not normally occur with this form of the disease.

In the U.S.A and some other countries, it appears that a similar virus that causes respiratory diseases can cause abortion following foetal death. If there is delay in expelling the dead foetus, an endometritis may be a sequel. The respiratory form of this disease in bulls can lead to damage within the testes that makes the animal infertile for months. Another variant of this virus occurs in Africa, causing a specific vaginitis in which there is a copious mucopurulent discharge but without vesicles. It causes epididymitis in bulls and apparently is always transmitted by mating.

There are other pathogenic viruses that have been implicated in causing death of the foetus and subsequent abortion. One is *bovine virus diarrhoea* or mucosal disease, and another epizootic bovine abortion, common in parts of North America and parts of Europe. Two bacterial infections, leptospirosis and salmonellosis that cause serious general signs of disease, will in the pregnant cow bring about the death of the foetus.

Protozoa

A Protozoa parasite, *Trichomonas foetus*, causes another venereal disease, passing from the bull to infect cows and heifers. This prevents conception and, if a pregnant animal becomes infected, will lead to abortion. The disease can be eradicated by employing artificial insemination, being sure to obtain the semen from healthy bulls. If this is done, infected cows will cure themselves; although, if there is a concomitant endometritis with other invading pathogens, the appropriate ancillary treatment must be given. Diagnosis of trichomoniasis is normally by the microscopic identification of the parasite in samples of vaginal mucus or a scraping from the bull's prepuce. Although drugs used to treat human trichomoniasis have been successfully used in bulls, it is generally considered safest to slaughter such animals.

Fungi

Occasionally the spores of a fungus that is found in mouldy hay, *Aspergillus*, are inhaled and, entering the bloodstream, infect the cotyledons of the cow's uterus and can in this manner cause the death of the foetus.

Sheep

There are three common causes of abortion in sheep:

1. Infection with the vibrio, *C. foetus intestinalis*, has already been mentioned, and it appears to be the commonest cause of abortion in intensively managed ewe flocks. Here losses may be as high as 20 per cent, occurring towards the end of pregnancy. Losses in the following year are greatly reduced because of the acquired immunity.
2. Enzootic abortion is caused by an infectious agent that belongs to the *Chlamydia* or PLV (psitticosis lymphogranuloma venereum) group, and on an initial infection of a flock, can cause 25-30 per cent abortions, again in the last 6 weeks of pregnancy. It is spread by ewes grazing where abortions have occurred or the pasture contaminated by vaginal discharges. It is not carried by the ram. An effective vaccine can be used to prevent or greatly reduce losses in a subsequent years.

3. An organism of the *Salmonella* group, *S. abortus-ovis* may from time to time cause abortions as well as illness in ewes from metritis and septicaemia. The disease is introduced by a bought-in animal who is a carrier. There are likely to be neonatal deaths in infected lambs and persistent diarrhoea causing later deaths with salmonellosis. The organism is sensitive to specific drugs, while a vaccine is available for the protection of healthy young animals.

From time to time, abortions in ewes, still-births and embryonic absorption may be caused by infection with *Toxoplasma gondii*. This is a microorganism that affects many species, including man, and locates in the central nervous system, muscles, the eyes and in the foetal cotyledons. Ewes become immune after infection and if fresh sheep are introduced into an affected flock, this should be done some time before mating to allow immunity to be acquired.

Sow

While there may be certain anatomical or physiological difficulties over reproduction with some sows, likely to be more marked with certain strains within breeds, infertility or abortion from infection is infrequent. In the U.S.A., *Brucella suis* has been widespread, causing inflammation of the testes (orchitis) in boars, abortion and sterility in sows and deaths in newly born piglets. The most effective way of dealing with this disease is to slaughter the whole herd as pig reach marketable weight and delay restocking, after thorough disinfection of the premises, for six months.

There are various virus diseases of pigs, e.g. swine fever, Aujeszky's disease, foot-and-mouth disease, swine influenza, that will prevent conception or interrupt gestation in sows, for they are serious generalized infections.

Bitch and cat

The commonest abnormality affecting reproduction in both the bitch and the cat is a hyperplasia or thickening of the wall of the uterus, often followed by infection, to produce a greatly distended womb. This stage is likely to produce toxaemia and signs of general illness, dullness, lack of appetite and raised temperature. In some instances, there will be a discharge of pus from the vagina.

This condition, especially in cats, is associated with non-breeding, since the effect of repeated cycles of progesterone/oestrogen secretion that occur during the normal cycle of females withheld from mating produces this thickening of the uterine wall with the formation of cysts in a fairly high proportion of older animals. It is generally necessary to perform hysterectomy (removal of the uterus).

Infertility from specific infection is rare, although two organisms are able to cause abortion. The first is confined to canines and is due to *Brucella canis*, infective also from the male, causing orchitis and epididymitis. Not seen in the U.K., it is common in the U.S.A., where infected bitches tend to abort at 45-55 days of pregnancy.

Toxoplasma gondii may occasionally cause abortion, stillbirth and neonatal deaths in both bitches and cats. It can be diagnosed from the multiple small soft nodules on the fresh placenta. Since this organism is transferable to humans, swift action to remove infected animals and careful disinfection of premises must be undertaken.

Other Causes of Infertility

The ability of any species to breed regularly is clearly desirable, but the dependence upon this function is greater in farm animals than in those of the companion animals. If a high-yielding dairy cow does not produce a calf every year, there is a loss of income. The Milk Marketing Board of England and Wales pointed out that in all four common dairy breeds those herds with calving intervals of about 375 days produced approximately the same quantity of milk per cow during the year, no matter in which month they calved.

In all breeds, herds that had calving intervals of over 400 days gave less milk. It has been calculated that every day of increase in the calving interval beyond 365 days results in financial loss of 77p, allowing for the costs of feeding. In other words, a single missed oestrus cost the farmer about £16. At this time the average dairy herd in England and Wales contained 44 cows and if its calving index was 395 days, the loss was approximately £1000 per years. Likewise, if a herd of sows does not produce an average of eight viable piglets twice yearly, or the lowland ewe flock a lambing percentage of 150 per cent or better, these farmers' incomes similarly suffer. These aims are more likely to be achieved if the following practical husbandry steps are followed.

Cattle

It has now come to be recognized that the modern dairy cow has a normal conception rate to first insemination of little more than 60 per cent. Those cows that do not conceive to a first service or insemination will likewise have a 60 per cent chance of conception at the end of the next heat period. Except with maiden heifers, dairy cows in North America and European countries are expected to be producing large quantities of milk at the time that efforts will be made to get them into calf again.

Management and conception

There is a continuing management problem because the identification of cows in oestrus is an indispensable step in making sure that the herd's calving index, i.e. the mean calving interval over all the milking cows, is kept down to approximately 365 days. There is often particular difficulty in detecting the heat period of maiden heifers at the age at which the first mating is to be made. Wherever the size of the enterprise merits the keeping of a bull, an effective method is to allow him to run with the heifers. Frequently, a beef bull—the Hereford is a favourite—is chosen, partly because of the smaller calf causing less trouble at birth, partly to obtain a higher price for the calf.

Where artificial insemination is used, there must be careful observation by the stockman to detect the signs of heat. As pro-oestrus ends, cows will show a variety of physical signs, swelling and, in light-coloured breeds, reddening of the vulva. Some cows will have a discharge of clear mucus from the vagina, but most will either attempt to mount other cows or will themselves stand still to permit mounting by other cows. Most oestrous activity occurs at night.

It is of the utmost importance that the stockman regularly observes the behaviour of all cows, and that the date of service for every cow be noted on the daily record sheet that is usually kept in the milking parlour. There are now readily available various designs of wall charts that make it quickly possible to ascertain calving dates and to mark the date at which individual cows must be carefully watched for a return to oestrus.

Electronic aids

Recent rapid increase in the use of microprocessors holds out the prospect that much important information concerning the management and recording of occurrences in each cow, can now be electronically stored and processed with the aid of small computers. Where herds have reached numbers in excess of 200, the cost effectiveness of having correlated information on production, health and reproduction readily available has already been demonstrated.

Functional Infertility

Occasionally cows will be encountered who exhibit abnormal patterns of oestrus as a result of hormonal imbalance. This may take the form of a continuing state of anoestrus—complete absence of heat periods. The cause is likely to be a persistent corpus luteum in the ovary. Most of these cows respond to treatment with the prostaglandin, $F_2\alpha$, or synthetic analogues, e.g. cloprostenol (Estrumate), dinoprost (Lutylase).

Another abnormality is the existence of what is called a cystic ovary. As a result of one or more follicles within the ovary not rupturing in the usual manner at the end of the oestrous cycle, there is a continuation of manifestations of heat. The cow will continue to stand to allow other cows to mount as well as often mounting other cows; the discharge from the vulva persists and there is slackening of the pelvic ligaments and elevation of the tail head. Such a syndrome may be called nymphomania. It is more likely to occur in heavy-milking strains, with cows after they have had their third or fourth calf, and during the early part of lactation as the cow comes up to the peak of her performance.

There is a suggestion that the abnormal quantity of circulating oestrogen responsible for this condition may be due to the high level of prolactin secretion from cows well fed and with high genetic capability for milk production and that this activity in the anterior pituitary may interfere with the secretion or release of sufficient luteinizing hormone to cause ovulation and normal corpus luteum formation, with its production of progesterone. This, in its turn, would inhibit follicle-stimulating hormone.

While treatment at one time was to rupture the cysts manually, with the consequent danger of adhesions developing in a proportion of instances, it is generally believed that injection of luteinizing hormone followed by progesterone is more effective. With the greater availability of luteinizing hormone releasing factor, this alone may be sufficient to get the cow cycling normally.

Embryonic loss

Surveys in many countries have shown that there is, with modern strains of high producing cows of whatever breed, up to a 30 per cent loss of embryos in the first few weeks after mating or insemination. The cause is uncertain but one suggestion is that this is due to the expression of deleterious or lethal recessive genes. With the rapid advancement of cytogenetics and the technique of examining the karyotype (the display of the animal's complement of chromosomes) the incidence of various aberrations has been determined.

Infertility and Nutrition

It has been shown that the energy intake of a high-producing cow during the first 80-100 days after calving, which is the period in which she is steadily increasing her milk output to reach her lactation peak, cannot match the energy being put out in the milk. In other words, she is bound to lose weight. A cow that is losing weight at too fast a rate during this time or is below her normal or optimal weight, is likely either not to show normal oestrus or not to ovulate. She may well stay in anoestrus, that is remain infertile until the lost weight is made up.

This emphasizes the importance of sufficient time, two months being sufficient for most cows, when she should be dry and fed increasing quantities of a diet containing a high proportion of digestible energy, balanced for protein and minerals. After calving, each cow should be fed an amount of a high energy ration calculated to be slightly more than the milk yield expected from each particular cow.

It has been shown that a long-continued deficiency of phosphorus either in absolute terms (less than 0.2 per cent of the diet) or relative to the intake of calcium if the latter is, as occasionally happens, too high, can induce infertility. Such a low effective intake of phosphorus is likely to be associated with diminished intake of digestible energy, since inappetance frequently accompanies this mineral deficiency.

Under exceptional conditions, a continued manganese deficiency may induce infertility. It occurs where there is a high pH of the soil, with excess calcium intake from legumes, which grow well under such conditions, and is accompanied by a deficiency in soil and pasture. Supplementation with the appropriate mineral—dicalcium phosphate, 56 g/h/day for a phosphorus deficiency and manganese sulphate, 4 g/h/day in the second instance—will eliminate these deficiencies.

Production Disease

Two of the three common metabolic disorders that are now frequently referred to as production diseases, viz. ketosis and grass tetany, will interrupt the normal reproduction rhythm. Ketosis is the clinical manifestation of the cow's inability to produce lactose in the udder from blood glucose. This is due to the shortage of oxaloacetate, a necessary substrate in the formation of lactose. This is in short supply because there has been interruption in the sufficiency of supply of the lower volatile fatty acids and glucose coming to the liver from the reticulo-rumen and the intestines. In other words, it is a more acute manifestation of a failure to provide enough digestible energy in the diet. Care in feeding will prevent ketosis, its treatment consisting in providing glucose by injection and a readily fermented material by mouth that will yield glucose, such as glycerol or propylene glycol. Corticosteroids are frequently given to supplement the supply from the adrenal cortex.

Sheep

As with cattle, there is well-documented evidence that there is a moderate level of embryonic death in ewes, probably about 12 per cent. Such ewes may well be successfully served at a succeeding heat period and carry a normal foetus to maturity.

As a result of grazing upon certain strains of subterranean clover in Australia (Dwalganap was a particularly dangerous strain) or of being given a diet containing a high proportion of some tetraploid strains of red clover (Hungaropoly), infertility can be a serious problem. This is due to an oestrogenic substance, genistin, that can lead to cystic degeneration of the endometrium. Avoidance of these strains and the vigilance of plant breeders in the production of newer high-yielding types of legumes, should minimize this danger in the future.

Sows

The farrowing rate as a result of a first service is between 70 and 80 per cent in most intensive pig production units in temperate climates. In the relatively very few enterprises where sows are allowed free-range and boars are run with them, the level of fertility may be expected to be higher.

The economics of pig production encourage the adoption of a system of three-week weaning in order to be more certain of getting two litters annually from each sow. With the older and more orthodox method of weaning at 8 weeks, the sow would show oestrus 4-5 days later, with a higher degree of probability that there would ensue a successful mating. If the system of weaning at three weeks is adopted, two factors of management will help to minimize the time before oestrus is shown. One is to be sure that the sow is fed a 16 per cent protein diet in generous amount and the second is to keep the sow within sound and smell of a boar.

Mare

The fertility of mares, particularly those of the various breeds of ponies, mating under natural conditions, is of the order of 90 per cent. Thoroughbred mares, kept under highly artificial conditions, entailing movement to stud premises for mating, have an average fertility of only 60 per cent. The irregularity of foaling in Thoroughbreds may be due to the infections already discussed, but management factors and a high rate of early embryonic mortality (approximately 19 per cent) play important parts in causing temporary infertility.

The chances of a successful mating are greater if mares are not covered until warmer spring weather and, where possible, the grazing of spring grass has wrought a conditioning effect. Lack of oestrus is the commonest cause of non-infectious infertility in the mare and is often due to lack of condition, i.e. being under weight due to inadequate diet or internal parasites. Bad environmental conditions may play a part too. A proportion of anoestrous mares have been shown to respond to infusion of prostaglandin into the uterus or by the simpler method of intramuscular injection.

Once a filly has had a foal, it is referred to as a 'brood mare' and is likely to be got into foal again as soon as possible. The question of whether a brood mare should be mated at the first or 'foal' heat period which occurs 9-10 days after giving birth to a foal, depends upon several considerations. The most important of these is to be sure that no pathogenic infection has become established in the uterus immediately following foaling, and that the uterus has properly involuted. If the mare is free of infection and is in good condition, she may be teased on the fourth and each successive day after foaling. It is likely that she will conceive at this first post-parturient oestrus.

Bitch and cat

There is remarkably little reliable information about the incidence and the nature of non-infectious infertility in the bitch and cat. Irregularity of oestrus increases with age, bitches over 5 years old having extended heat periods or failing to reproduce altogether. When there is failure of an otherwise normal young bitch or queen to come into oestrus, injections of follicle-stimulating hormone are given. Vaginal smears should be examined and, when the end of pro-oestrus is shown, an injection of luteinizing hormone may permit successful mating.

7

Horses and Mules

The proper evaluation and selection of either purebred or grade draft animals is a much more complicated job than that of properly evaluating other farm animals. In addition to the conformation, quality, and condition of the horse or mule, the buyer or judge must also consider the feet, legs, action, wind, and temperament. The importance of these last items is reflected in the old sayings "No foot—no horse" and "The feet, legs, and action are half the horse."

To properly evaluate draft animals one must first learn the proper names for the different parts, and then he must consider the purpose of work stock and how they accomplish their purpose. Draft horses and mules are designed principally to pull more or less heavy loads at a medium to slow gait. Practically all of the power for this pull is generated in the rear quarters of the horse and mule.

The pull is exerted almost entirely through the rear feet with the front feet serving mostly to support the front part of the animal as would a set of wheels. From the rear feet the force is transmitted through the rear legs, loin, back, and shoulders into the collar. These facts warrant the drawing of several conclusions:

1. The feet of a draft animal must not only be sound but should also be large so that they can obtain maximum grip on the ground.
2. The bone of the draft animal must be strong and durable and the legs must be placed or "set" properly.
3. The hocks must be broad, deep, and clean because these are the levers through which the power, generated in the muscles of the rear quarters, is transmitted to the feet when pulling.

4. The gaskins, quarters, thighs and croup of the animal must be heavily muscled, since these generate the pulling power.
5. The loin and back must be short, broad, and heavily muscled in order to carry the thrust from the rear quarters to the shoulder.
6. The shoulders must be sloping and clean cut so as to give a good seat to the collar and permit an alert carriage of head and neck and a long, easy stride.
7. The middle should be sufficiently deep and roomy to provide enough capacity for feed, especially pasture and roughage, so that the work animal can maintain his condition with a minimum of expense for concentrates.
8. The chest must be deep and wide so as to provide sufficient lung capacity to take care of the needs of the animal while working at or near top capacity.
9. The pasterns, especially the front ones, must slope at approximately a 45-degree angle, since the front feet are raised higher and, consequently, strike the ground harder than the rear feet. The angle of the pastern absorbs this shock and, thereby, tends to prevent ring-bones, splints, side-bones and other blemishes and unsoundnesses caused by excessive and repeated shock.
10. The horse or mule must be willing and alert since a balky or sluggish draft animal will waste both his time and that of the driver.

One of the most difficult things for beginners to learn is the proper placement of feet and legs. Animals are seldom seen with all four legs squarely in place. Show animals having faulty set to legs or hocks are usually placed so as to make these defects less obvious. Once the proper placement of feet and legs is learned, however, it is relatively easy to spot defects. As an aid to learning the correct placement for the feet and legs of a horse or mule study Figure, which shows both the correct placement and the most common deviations from this.

Ideal Draft Animal

Even though horses and mules do not closely resemble each other, they serve the same purpose; their ideals in size, conformation, quality, and action are very similar. The main difference lies in the closeness to which each approaches this ideal. Some mule men contend that a mule that looks too much like a horse lacks the durability expected of a mule. There is some truth in this argument. However, in both the sale ring and the show ring the mule is measured against much the same standard of perfection as the horse. He is usually most deficient in quality of head; muscling over the back, loin, and croup; fullness in the rear quarters; size and quality of feet and bone; and set of hind legs.

Size

The ideal size for a draft animal will vary with the section of the country, the size of the farm, and the job that is to be done. The extra-large, clumsy horse that was popular in the North some 20 years ago, has now been replaced with a 16-hand (a "hand" is four inches), 1600-pound horse that is no taller from the sole of his foot to his chest floor than from his chest floor to the top of his withers. This newer type is more active, handier with its feet, and easier to keep fit.

Southerners prefer even lighter horses and consider a 1000 to 1400 pound horse to be sufficiently large. Mules vary in weight all the way from the 12-hand, 600-pound pit-mining mule to the 17-hand, 1600-pound draft mule. Large mules are usually worth more money than the smaller ones.

Head and Neck

The head is a good index of the animal's quality and should be clean cut, tapering gradually from the eyes to the poll and from the eyes to the nostrils. It should be neither large and coarse nor small and ultrarefined, but should closely approximate the length of the animal's shoulders. The eyes should be large, set wide apart, clear and quiet. Horses' ears should be of medium size and texture and should be carried at an alert angle. Mules' ears, while larger than the horse's should be relatively trim and fine. The union of the head and neck, known as the "throat latch," should be clean-cut or free from thickness and meatiness. The jaws should be widespread to prevent choking as the animal flexes his neck while pulling.

The neck should be tapering, supple, and of moderate length. Short, stubby necks usually are found on horses that are hard to guide and hard to fit with a collar. Mules are inclined toward "ewe" necks.

Shoulders

The shoulders should be well laid-in at their top, blending smoothly into the withers. The shoulder should have approximately a 45- degree slope and a clean-cut, well-defined collar bed. Steep shoulders mean a low carriage of head and neck and consequently a short, stubby stride. They are also more apt to become blemished under hard work.

Body

The draft animal should be short and heavily muscled in his neck and loin, deep and broad in his chest, well sprung in his rib so as to have a deep, round middle, and he should be deep or well let-down in his hind flank. These characteristics insure ample lung and stomach capacity as well as a strong top for heavy pulls. Light-middled horses and mules are hard keepers. Animals with sharp backs and narrow lions lack the necessary muscling to stand up under heavy work.

Rear Quarters

The hindquarters of the draft animal generate most of the pulling power. They should therefore be wide, deep, and heavily muscled. The croup should be long, broad, and gently sloping. The thighs should be wide, deep, and heavily muscled. The gaskins and stifle should show heavy, bulging muscling. The mule is most commonly deficient in the rear quarters.

Feet, Legs, and Action

The proper placement of feet and legs has already been discussed. The feet should be large, round, sloping from front to rear, and wide at the heels. The horn of the hoof should be dense, smooth, and free from cracks. The rear feet are not as side at the heel as are the front feet. While most mules have relatively small, narrow feet, larger feet with quality are preferred.

The pasterns should slope at approximately a 45-degree angle and have sufficient length and elasticity to absorb the shock and to permit an easy gait. Short, upright pasterns go with a jerky gait and unsoundnesses, especially of the front pasterns and legs.

The cannon bones are the best place to observe quality of bone. The bone should be of medium size, dense, and flat. Knees should be deep from front to rear, wide as viewed from the front, and tapering gradually into the leg.

The hock is of outstanding importance since this is the lever used to transmit the power of the rear quarters in propelling the animal forward. The hock should be wide from front to rear, deep from top to bottom, and wide at the front. It should be clean-cut and free from blemishes and unsoundnesses.

The draft animal should have a long, straight, snappy yet easy stride. He should lift his feet high enough to clear obstacles, but not so high as to be wasteful of energy. Throwing the feet outward as they are moved forward is called "paddling". Exaggerated paddling in high-going horses is called "winging". "Interfering" is striking one foot against the other as it is moved forward. Moving forelegs around each other and planting them in a single, straight line is called "winding" or "rope-walking." Striking a front shoe or foot with a rear foot is called "forging." "Rolling" is shifting of weight from side to side to keep balance—a defect found especially in excessively wide-chested horses. "Pounding" is hitting the ground too hard, whereas a quick, high, but short stride is described as being "trappy." Traveling wide at the hocks is a serious fault, since an animal so affected springs out at the hocks under heavy pull and punches himself in the belly with his stifle at the trot.

Common Blemishes and Unsoundnesses

A *blemish* is an imperfection or injury not serious enough to interfere with the serviceability of the animal. An *unsoundness* is an imperfection of form or function that is caused by inheritance, injury, overwork, or misuse and that interfere with the serviceability or usefulness of the animal in a way that greatly lowers his value. Work stock are usually sold with or without guarantees as to soundness as follows:

1. "Sound"—guaranteed free from any unsoundness or serious blemishes.
2. "Serviceably sound"—showing only blemishes or unsoundnesses that do not affect his usefulness.
3. "At the halter"—no guarantee as to soundness, disposition, or any other characteristic.

Unsoundnesses vary as to their effect on the usefulness of a horse or mule. It is usually accepted that the following constitute show-ring disqualifications: lameness, blindness, bone spavin, stifled, stringhalt, ringbone, one testicle or abnormal testicles in a stallion, and bad wind.

The following defects are recognized as ground for more or less serious discrimination: sidebone, bog spavin, thoropin, capped hock, cocked ankle, poll evil, filled hock, curb, fistula, umbilical rupture, and stocked ankles.

Definitions of the more common blemishes and unsoundnesses are given:

Bone spavin—a bony growth usually found on the inside lower part of the hock joint.

Bog spavin—a soft swelling located at the front inside area of the hock.

Thoropin—a soft swelling similar to a bog spavin but located in the depression just in front of the point of the hock. Pressure on one side will cause the swelling to bulge out on the other side.

Curb—a swelling at the rear of and toward the bottom of the hock.

Ringbone—a bony growth around part or all of a pastern.

Sidebone—a prominence and hardness at the hoofhead caused by ossification of the lateral cartilage.

Splint—a bony growth lying along the inside of the front cannon bone below the knee.

Stifled—dislocation of the patella of the stifle joint; usually incurable and crippling.

Stringhalt—a nervous disease resulting in a jerky, abnormally-high action of the hocks.

Fistula—a deep seated abscess at the withers.

Poll evil—similar to fistula but located at the poll.

Heaves—a respiratory disease characterized by wheezy and jerky breathing and a short hollow cough.

Blindness—a result of injury, infection, or "moon blindness" causing loss of sight in one or both eyes.

Capped hock—a prominence at the point of the hock usually caused by bruising.

Cocked ankle—usually found on rear legs with unusually steep pasterns caused by shortening or inflammation of the tendons and resulting in a short, stubby and frequent stumbling.

Market Classes and Grades of Horses and Mules

There are no up-to-date official market classes and grades of horses and mules. They vary from market to market and from year to year. The following represents an average classification for the country as a whole.

Draft Horses

Draft horses surpass the other classes of work animals in conformation, weight, and quality. They are deep-bodied, short-legged, thick, heavily-muscled, and of good quality.

Chunks

These are similar to draft horses, having approximately the same conformation and quality, but less size. They are used principally for farm work.

Wagon Horses

These are similar to chunks in size, but are somewhat more leggy and possess more quality and speed. They are used principally in cities on milk, bakery, and other delivery wagons.

Driving Horses

The demand for driving horses has been practically eliminated by motor vehicles. The remaining demand is principally for pleasure and show purposes. Both outlets expect and will pay for quality. Roadsters and principally of Standardbred breeding and possess quality and speed. Heavy harness horses are principally of American Saddle Horse or Hackney breeding. They are a somewhat more stylish horse than the roadster and possess higher but shorter action. They are, therefore, not so fast as the roadster.

Saddle Horses

These vary in quality from the western bronco to the finest of 5-gaited saddle horses, and in size from the upper pony limit of 14.2 hands to the large, upstanding hunter of 17.2 or better. Light hunters and jumpers are usually of Thoroughbred breeding, whereas heavy hunters and jumpers often carry a cross of Percheron blood.

Ponies

This class arbitrarily includes anything under 14.2 hands in height. They vary from the chunky, rather plain-legged children's pet, to the clean-cut, stylish show pony.

Classes and Grades of Mules

Mules are classified according to their use and graded according to their quality and value. A short description of each class follows:

Draft mules are the largest of all mules and are used for teaming, contracting jobs, and lumbering. These should be of drafty type, good quality; and straight and snappy action.

Farm mules are usually of somewhat poorer type, quality, and finish than are draft mules. They are purchased for use as farm work stock principally in the central and southern states. Mare mules are preferred.

Sugar mules are used on southern sugar plantations. They are between the draft and cotton mules in size, type, and quality. Mare mules are preferred because of their higher quality and more active dispositions.

Cotton mules are purchased for use on the cotton plantations of the South. They are definitely lighter and less drafty in type than the sugar mule. The present trends in southern farming call for larger and better mules than were used a number of years ago.

Mining mules vary greatly in size and weight according to the type of mine work they are to do. They should be of compact, drafty type. Geldings are preferred because of their more sluggish dispositions. Mules are well adapted to use in mines because they are quieter than ponies and less apt to be injured by misuse.

Factors Affecting Marketing Value of Horses and Mules

Class. The market class for which an animal can qualify will determine to a large extent his value. It can be seen that since 1935 saddle horses of even medium quality have outsold the average draft horse, wagon horse, or chunk.

Age. The value of a horse or mule also depends on its age since they may be either too young to work or too old to have much serviceable life left.

Sex. Mares are preferred to geldings wherever the buyer plans to raise foals for replacements or for sale. Mare mules are also preferred, except in mines, because of their higher quality and more alert, active dispositions.

Conformation. The conformation of a horse or mule greatly affects its serviceability and therefore its value. Narrow, upstanding, light-muscled draft horses sell at a considerable discount. So do low-headed, coarse, stubby saddle horses.

Quality. Quality of bone and feet is especially important since it is an indication of durability. General quality is closely related to price.

Colour. Preferences differ, but generally speaking the solid and darker colours are preferred. In teams the colours should be matched.

Temperament. Any evidence of vices or skittishness detracts from the value of an animal. However, a spirited and energetic animal of tractable disposition is preferred.

Training. The average buyer wants a well-trained animal.

Condition. Fat covers a multitude of defects. It also indicates that the animal is healthy and has been well cared for.

Style. This is especially important in saddle horses. A little work in grooming and trimming often pays big dividends.

Action. The action of a horse or mule is closely related to its serviceability. Those with short, low, sluggish, or crooked action can do less work, give a poor ride, and often become unsound due to physical defects that cause undue strain on joints or bones as well as poor action while so doing.

Soundness. An unsound or even a blemished animal should sell at a considerable discount since most unsoundnesses affect an animal's usefulness in a greater or lesser degree.

8

TRANSGENIC PIGS

Domestication of mammals has been an old and profitable business of man. It has been recorded in prehistoric period also. The domesticated mammals, in olden days, were used either for milk, traveling or for meat. There is a long list of animals domesticated by the man. These mammals help the man in various ways. Some of the common mammals which are domesticated by the man are cow, ox, deer, dogs, cats, buffaloes, elephants, horses, donkeys and pigs. Today a number of industries are base on animals and their by-products. Thus these animals are providing handsome jobs to unemployed educated youngmen. Sheeps, goats ans swines are more successful in acilmatising themselves in each and every environment so the industries based on these animals are always in profit and they are preferred by a large number of people. The rearing and development of sheep, goat and swine requires less economies and technology whereas the rate of production is high and duration of maturity is much less as compared with another mammal.

Rearing, development and breeding of swine is known as *piggery*. It is one of the most common and desired industry in developed countries and is gaining momentum in developing countries like India. Pig rearing has never been a new thing for Indian people, but its raising and production has always been in primitive stage. There is no scientific planning and investment of money only because of the reason that it is in the hands of poor and uneducated persons. The higher class of people, educated students and economically sound parties did not show their interest in formation of pig houses and development of a piggery.

The Country Pig

The common Indian pigs are most neglected, scrub animals without any marked characteristic features. They are not paid proper attention and food for their development hence they do not get a fair chance to grow into economical animals and compete with them. These swines are small, black and produce small litters. The meat is also not up to the mark and quite often they are infested with a variety of worms and diseases. They grow slower and die soon. The common Indian pigs have higher fat contents so they are used for medicinal purposes and the flesh is not tasty.

Advantages of pig Production

1. Pig forming requires less money, space and technology.
2. The pigs are developed in comparatively shorter period and with minimum expenditure. They pay the return in the shortest possible time as compared with any other form animals.
3. The housing and equipments are not costly
4. They do not require much labour and attention as compared with any other form animal.
5. The retrun of money is always in a handsome amount as compared with dairy and poultry.
6. The pigs grow faster than any other animal.

Efficiency in Park Production

The profit in production of the pig depends upon the efficiency of the grower in production of the pig and its marketing. He must have a look over the rate of growth, amount of feed eaten and quality of grains used in the feed. The supplementation of vitamins, minerals, antibiotics and proteins in the feed helps in developing the swine faster and such as swine always fetch a good amount of money.

Since the hogs and swines are subjected to a large number of parasites and diseases proper case is to be taken against these diseases.

The swine used in the piggery should be of an improved quality and she must have a good breeding capacity. At the same time marketing of the pig also plays an important role in its economics.

Selection of Breeds

In establishing a piggery the selection of breed plays an important role. It depends on the will of the grower as what type of pig he wants to grow. The profit and loss depends mostly on the selection of the pig. Some of the common breeds aclimatised in India are given below. These breed can be divided into two major groups.

1. The English Class
2. The American Class

The English Class

This class of breed generally includes the pig of English origin. They are well aclimatised in Indian environment and are used for improving the race. Some of the common English breeds are :

(a) *The Large White Yorkshire*. It is an English breed but well established in U.S.A., Canada, India, Ireland and countries of Indian sub-continents. They are used for upgrading the Indian breed. These are white, big in size long and bulky with a long thin and forwardly inclined ears. They measure 350-400 kg.

(b) *Middle White Yorkshire*. A English cross breed boar developed by crossing the white large with Yorkshire extraction. It is a high class bred famous for good quality of meat. It has an early maturing and good recovery. It converts the food into meat in large ratio. These are white, large sized, with a long back and level. They measure about 270 to 380 kg.

Berkshire

This is the oldest breed of swine now established in Australia, Newzeland and Berkshire. It is famous for high yield and is used in upgrading the Indian breed. These can be recognised by its black colour and white patches on the feet, head and tail. The head is short and face is blunt. They weigh 280-300 kg.

American Breed

The American breeds are equally good for upgrading the Indian races and meat production as well. They can be aclimatised easily in Indian environment and are widely used in all parts of India. Some of the common breeds are:

Chester White

A native of Pensylvania U.S.A. is a cross breed of English white Yorkshire with Cheshire and Lincohnshire breeds. These are white in colour and produce big litters. The litters develop fast and reach maturity very soon they measure about 400 kg.

Duroc

Red coloured with white shade in colour. The colour may vary from golden to dark red. They develop fast and produce big litters. They have high milking capacity. These are used in cross breeding weigh about 300 kg.

Hampshire

These are black pigs with white best encircring the body and fornt legs. Head and tail are black, ears straight and erected. Legs are short and produce good quantity of milk and meat as well.

Besides these a variety of porks are found which are equally good in amount of meat and its quality but require more attention. These breeds are Poland, China, Tamworth and Wessex saddleback etc. Day by day improved varieties are being produced which mature early and give flavoured quality of meat in large amount.

Feeding and Management of the Herd

The profit or loss of a pigger is determined on the basis of the total net gain from the piggery. This gain is calculated on the basis of the number of pits marketed. The number of pig produced in the herd depends on a variety of factors and feeding is one of them. Food feeding of the male boar and the sow is solely responsible for producing a big litter. A protein rich diet keeps the male active and smart. It produces a good quantity of sperm with a large number of viable motile sperms, in the same way a healthy female produces a large number of eggs and they are fertilized perfectly. Such a sow produces healthy litter with maximum viability and minimum mortality. Such a sow produces less number of abnormal pigs. The diet of a lactating female is little different with the same given to the male.

The pigs have a very simple digestive system without much modifications and complications, so they require a good and protein rich diet. They are unable to digest more fibrous food but fibrous food up to a limited extent is also necessary for their proper development. A protein rich food helps the female in producing more and more milk and this effects the health of the body sow up to great extent. A healthy baby sow changes the food quickly and starts feeding on grains and fodder where as a ill fed baby sow continues on mother milk for a longer period.

The feed of a sow should have low fibre contents such as cereal grains and their byproducts. It should have proper proportion of minerals, vitamins, medicines, and antibiotics along with the protein. It is to be in a measured quantity, which can keep a pig fast growing, healthy and strong but at the same time should not be much high in fat contents because enough of fat in a sow makes the meat of low quality. There should be a limited ratio of fat and flesh. The balanced diet of a swine comprises of the following ingradients :

Maize, ground barley or grain jowar = 65-75%
Ground wheat or oat = 15%
Meat scrap = 5-7%
Soya meal = 6-10%
Minerals = .5-1%
Salt = 0.5%

If such a balanced diet is given to a male swinc he can be ready and it for service after 8 months whereas a female gets matured in 9 months. It is not advised to use a male in early stage, for better and fruitful results he should be used after one year and that too not daily. He must be given rest at least for 3 days before his use and in the same way the female should not be allowed to male just after her first cycle, she must be spared for 2-3 cycles, i.e., 2-3 months after her first cycle. This cause full development of the uterus and ova and gives better result in days to come. The maturation of male and female depends upon the quality and quantity of the food, they are fed with.

The food of a meat quality of sow varies much from the food of a pregnant or milking sow they require more protein diet as compared with any other normal sow.

Gestation Period

The sow have a heat period of about 40-65 hrs. and the best period of their mating and population is the second half period during the heat period. A pig can easily be recognised during this stage because of her actions. She may mount other swines in the herd and will remain rest less and will not eat. Her appetite is lost. She can be recongnised by examination her vulva which becomes enlarged and congested but this can be done by expert breeders only. The cycle repeats after every third week, otherwise they have gestation period of 114 days on an average which may range from 112-115 days.

Artificial Insemination

Artificial insemination in swines plays a vital role in the development of piggery. In such a condition the boar of a good health and breed is allowed to mate a dummy female with pulsating vagina and the semen is collected in the glass vials. A boar is given at least three days rest after first ejaculation so he can serve only twice a week. The amount of sperms produce varies from 200-250 ml per boar which is kept in freezed condition after diluting with 6% glucose soln. The viability of sperms is 100% for the first 24 hrs after that the viability declines and the chance of fertilizing an egg is reduced to only 50% if such a frozen semen is used after three days. For good litter production a sow is crossed twice after an interval of 8 hrs. This gives good result as the chance of fertilizing an egg is doubled.

In Indian artificial inseminations in swine is not done on large scale because the number of piggeries are not much and if some of them are interested in having a piggery farming they prefer to have a boar also. This ceases the scope of A_1 in sows. Here are some practical problems associated with the artificial insemination of the swine such s the sperms have high mortality and poor ability of frozen sperms. The sow have small vagina which does not exhibit the visual symptoms of heat and they too show poor heat detections.

The sows in a herd have different days of heat so they can be managed by the boar.

The scientists in England have developed a new chemical which is fed to the female swine regularly and till the date it is fed to the sow she does not come into heat and the day the dose is checked the sow comes in heat. This has become a boon for piggery farming. The breeders check the heat period chemically and allow all the females of the herd to come in heat on same day. This helps in A_1 and all the females give birth to the hogs on the calculated day. This provides the breeder with a benefit of arranging and managing the females of same category. A particular type of bed. Feed, heat, water, mineral, vitamins and aids is given to the female during her pregnancy. This saves a breeder from arranging various types of beds, feeds, aids and at the same time large number of baby pigs are obtained which are marketed in a lot and the profit is obtained in a handsome amount. These things are still needed in India to improve the piggery farming.

The baby pig is given a good nutritive diet to develop fast and attain good size. Fatty diet is given only at certain intervals and after recommendation of the doctors. The well developed hog is now send to slaughter house or market. The slaughter of a pig is done after starving the pig for 24 hrs. This gives a good and standard product.

Growth of Young

For the good growth of young ones, supplementary feed should be given after 25 day by creep feeding. It should be kept in mind that sows fed on synthetic diet may not be allowed to become much fatty otherwise the size of the litter would be smaller. The good growth in the early developmental stages plays very significant role for the development in length, muscle, weight of the pits, so up to the age of 25 days young pigs should be fed on highly nutritive and easily digestible diet. The young pigs, with the weight of 50 pounds feeding on less nutritive diet, have good ability of fast growth to attain the maximum weight provided a good nutritive diet is given to them.

Proportional Growth of the Body

The proportional growth of the body of pigs varies with the age i.e.,the head and the legs are larger in comparison to the body but the age, the body grows very fast as a result the muscles of thigh become concave. Such growth is found more in middle white pig in comparison to large white pig. It is very useful to have an idea about the change in the weight of the developing pigs and a proper control on that change.

The growth in pigs runs from the cranium towards backwards and from the tail forwards which meet in the lumber vertebrae as a result the loin region grows very fast followed by the pelvis and the thorax than the neck. The head grows very slowly, it is advisable that the pigs in early stages should be allowed to fed on poor diet due to which early developing parts, as head and legs would grow very slowly and if later given highly nutritive diet the parts which grow later i.e., loin would grow very fast and the carcass with high proportion of fat is produced. In the young pigs the fat is soft and in the older ones it becomes firmer when growth rate is very fast and fat is synthesized from the carbohydrates.

Slaughter of Pigs

Prior to the killing, the pigs should be kept on starvation for 24 hours and given complete rest to get standard product. The slaughtering of pig is carried out by making it unconscious by a hard stroke given on the head, and piercing a double edged knife in the neck to shed the blood out of its jugular veins. Now carcass is washed, cleaned well in hot water and cut open to separate the various parts for different preparations.

PRODUCTS OF PIGGERY

Pork

The flesh of pig is known as pork in general and the fleshes obtained from different parts of the body have been given different name e.g., Bacon obtained from the back and sides and Ham from the back of the thigh. According to the data produced by the Directorate of Marketing and inspection, Government of India the production of pork is 5 percent of total production of meat in India.

Bristles

The wiry and stiff haris of the pigs, hogs and wild boars are known as bristles and they are obtained from the back and neck. Short bristles are obtained from the flanks and belly of the animal. The bristles obtained from the living pigs are superior in quality than those of slaughtered ones. The rough and coars bristles are generally used for varnish work and painting brushes. The main bristle producing areas are Uttar Pradesh, Madhya Pradesh, and Punjab. The principal trading centres are Kanpur and Jabalpur but 70 percent of the total bristle export is being made from Kanpur.

Two types of bristles viz., *Desi bristles* obtained from pigs of Uttar Pradesh and Madhya Pradesh, and *Darjeeling bristles*, obtained from Himalayan foot hill and Darjeeling district. The bristles of three colours are usually found viz., white, grey and black.

The important bristle markets in the country are at Agra, Allahabad, Azamgarh, Faizabad, Jaunpur, Amaraoti, Nagpur, Santhal Parganas, Caluctta and Kakinada.

Mumbai is the biggest port to export the bristles worth millions of dollars to U.S.A., U.K., Germany and Japan. Indian Standard Institute, New Delhi standardizes the bristles and provides *agmark*. Only the properly graded bristles under 'Bristle Grading and Marketing (amendment) Rules-1962' are permitted for export purposes.

Sausages

Sausages are prepared by fresh minced pork, free from bone and skin. For the preparation of sausages usually shoulder piece, ham and bacon are preferred. The sausages are prepared by washing, cooking and mixing the pork with spices such as white pepper and paprika to make it delicious.

Lard

The fat of pig, squeezed from the body tissue is termed as lard. For the preparation of lard, carcasses are cut into pieces, minced, boiled over a furnace and the fat is removed-carefully when it is boiling hot. Lard is used as a fine cooking medium and in the manufacture of soaps, lubricants, greases, candles and water proof materials.

Other Uses

The most important pharmaceuticals derived from thyroid, pituitary and pancereas of pigs are pepsin, thyroxin, pitutrin, insulin, liver extract, testesteron etc. The pig toe-nails are used for making tobacco fertilizer, plaster and other plastic materials. The blood is used as food for livestock and poultry and also as a manure.

Diseases and Control

The swine production suffer heavy loss due to diseases and parasites. These parasite kill the baby pigs and check proper growth and development of the pig as adult. They damage about 60-65% of the total pigs produce, either directly or indirectly. Their control is a major factor in swine production.

Most of the diseases can be controlled by applying preventive measures and proper sanitation. Over crowding, mismanagement, roaming of pigs in open places should be checked. Vaccination and medication at regular intervals helps in preventing the diseases.

In India swines are subjected to various diseases like, plague, flue, fever, pox, foot and mouth diseases, cholera, navel ill and dysentery and tuberculosis etc. These diseases are contageous diseases and can be checked by proper sanitation and care.

The infected pig becomes weak, looses its weight, the loss in appetite and vigour is well marked. He may sit or stand alone in an unusual manner. The colour of urine and faecal matter changes and some times it is supplemented with mucous and blood also. The colour may be red, green or black. Coughing and eye and nasal discharge is well marked in cold and flue cases. They stop feeding and go for water quite often. Parasites also play a vital role in swine business. The common parasites are round worm, hook worm, type worms, lungworm and mange. Ticks and mites, flea, mosquitoes, lice and bugs are common ectoparasites on pigs which may cause skin disease and itch.

These worms and ecto and endo parasites are reduced in number if proper care is taken in the management of a pig house, ventilation, sanitation and space have their role in minimising the parasites. These houses should be cleaned 2 sprayed with DDT, BHC or Gamexene.

Production of Transgenic Pigs by DNA Microinjection

Transgenesis includes a number of steps that are common to all the species discussed in this volume: superovulation, embryo recovery, embryo microinjection (or another method of transferring DNA), and embryo transfer to a recipient animal for gestation to term. Livestock species such as the pig can present special problems because of their size and housing requirements but they may have special advantages, such as litter size (12–14 piglets). The experimental manipulation of pigs for the production of transgenics is very much like that for mice, with some key differences that are primarily logistical in nature. We will try to point these out and to make recommendations where possible.

Transgenic pigs are key players in the area of biomedical models of human disease, and hold the promise of unlimited organs for transplant to humans. Refinements based originally on transgenic technology such as cloning and knock-out strategies bring the pig to the forefront of biomedical research. Man may live longer with pig parts substituting for failing human organs. The knowledge gained from pigs will bring many advances to human medicine. The techniques described below have been used to make transgenic pigs, and many of them can be used in other more recently developed techniques, such as cloning.

In Vivo Produced Embryos

In vivo produced embryos will always have the greatest viability and thus, almost all experiments have used fertilized embryos from donor females. In our laboratory, we have synchronized and superovulated prepubertal female pigs, flushed the embryos from the reproductive tract, and proceeded to manipulate the embryos. Surviving embryos were then transferred to one or two of the best donors for gestation to term. Synchronized, superovulated flushed donors serve as recipients, with very good success. They have been screened for their response (number and quality of embryos) and their ovaries have been evaluated prior to transfer. In terms of viability, in vivo produced embryos should always have the highest viability compared to in vitro produced embryos. Improvements in in vitro procedures will narrow the gap between in vitro and in vivo embryos, but will probably never close it.

In Vitro Produced Embryos

Matured porcine oocytes can be purchased from a number of commercial sources. These oocytes can be brought into the laboratory and subjected to in vitro fertilization to provide embryos for microinjection. However, there are some problems. First, in vitro produced embryos have a lower viability. One might expect that this would be nicely compensated by transferring more embryos to each recipient, but this is not always the case. The second problem, polyspermy, provides another stumbling block in the use of in vitro produced embryos. The Petters' laboratory and many others have worked extensively on these problems and still they remain largely unresolved. Two recent papers provide us with some indication of the magnitude of the problem. In one case, only 20% of the oocytes were normally fertilized, the problem being a combination of low fertilization rate (60%) and high polyspermy rate (67% of fertilized oocytes). In the second case, similar results were obtained. A slightly increased fertilization rate (70%) and a lower polyspermy rate were reported (53%) leaving one-third of the oocytes normally fertilized. With practice, it may be possible to separate unfertilized from fertilized oocytes, this leaves the polyspermic (50–60%) and normal oocytes that will be subjected to centrifugation and probably microinjected. At least twice as many embryos may have to be microinjected in order to produce enough embryos for transfer. With some sort of compensation for the predicted lower viability, these embryos can be transferred to recipients. This approach has a number of potential advantages: (i) not as many animals are needed because embryo donors are not required; (ii) surgical recovery of embryos is not required. Disadvantages may include: (i) more embryos may have to be injected because of lower viability and decreased number of normally fertilized embryos; (ii) recipients may be suboptimal and so pregnancy rate might suffer. Since the advent of cloning, this technique can be combined with transgenesis by using in vitro matured oocytes and somatic cells that have been genetically modified.

PROTOCOL FOR IN VITRO PRODUCTION OF PIG EMBRYOS

Media, Solutions and Reagents

There are two media systems currently available for use for the in vitro production of pig embryos: the standard system and the PPM (Purdue Porcine Media, developed by Rebecca Krisher) system. The details of media components for all media needed for each step in each system are given below.

Procedure	*PPM media system*	*Standard media system*
Maturation	PPMmat	TCM 199
Fertilization	PPMfert	mTBM
	Synthetic oviductal fluid (SOF) HEPES	SOF HEPES
Sperm wash	D-PBS	Sperm wash medium
	Percoll (45% and 90%)	D-PBS
	Percoll (45% and 90%)	
In vitro culture	PPM 1, PPM2	NCSU23

TCM1 99 oocyte maturation medium

Reagent	*Defined*	*Undefined*
TCM199	9.5 ml	8.5
Polyvinyl alcohol	0.01 g	–
PFF	–	1.0 ml
Glucose (3.05 mM; 0.5496 g/10 ml TCM199)	100 μl	100 μl
Pyruvate (0.91 mM; 0.05 g/5 ml TCM199)	100 μl	100 μl
PSA	100 μl	100 μl
Cysteine (0.5 mM; 0.05 g/5 ml TCM199)	100 μl	100 μl
pLH (porcine luteinizing hormone; 0.01 U/ml)	50 μl	50 μl
pFSH (porcine follicle stimulating hormone; 0.01 U/ml)	50 μl	50 μl
EGF (epidermal growth factor, 50 ng/ml; 0.1 mg/10 ml D-PBS)	10 μl	10 μl

Add reagents to TCM199 the morning of oocyte collection. Filter, make wells and place wells and medium in the incubator.

In vitro fertilization medium (mTBM)

mTBM Stock (modified Tris-buffered medium)

Reagent	*mM*	*g/100 ml*
NaCl	113.1	0.6611
KCl	3.0	0.0224
$CaCl_2 \cdot 2H_2O$	7.5	0.1102
Tris	20.0	0.2423
Glucose	11.0	0.1982
Na-pyruvate	5.0	0.0550

Filter. After preparation the pH should be about 10. Do not adjust. Store at 4°C. Good for 2 weeks.

mTBM working solution

- Combine 9.9 ml mTBM stock, 0.004 g caffeine (2 mM), 100 μl PSA (penicillin/streptomycin/amphotercin, an antibiotic antimycotic) and 0.02 g fraction V BSA. Filter and use.

Sperm wash medium

D-PBS w/o $CaCl_2$

- Make D-PBS according to directions on packet, omitting the $CaCl_2$. Make 1 l and adjust pH to 7.2–7.4. Filter. Store at 4°C. Good for 3 months.

Sperm wash medium working solution

- Add 0.05 g fraction V BSA and 500 μl PSA to 50 ml D-PBS.

Percoll

To make 90% Percoll solution, combine 45 ml Percoll (Sigma) with 5 ml 10 × stock of modified sperm TL.

10x stock modified sperm TL

Chemical	*g/100 ml*
KCl	0.230
NaH_2PO_4	0.035
NaCl	4.675
HEPES	2.380
Adjust pH to 7.3	

To this 50 ml of 90% Percoll, add:

Chemical	*Per 50 ml*
$CaCl_2$	14.5 mg
$MgCl_2 \cdot 6H_2O$	4.0 mg
Lactic acid	0.184 ml
$NaHCO_3$	104.5 mg

Synthetic oviductal fluid (SOF) HEPES medium

Stock A (base) 10×; 3 months expiration

Reagent	*mM*	*g/100 ml*	*g/200 ml*	*g/500 ml*	*g/1,000ml*
NaCl	99.7	5.827	11.654	29.135	58.270
KCl	7.16	0.534	1.068	2.670	5.340
KH_2PO_4	1.19	0.162	0.324	0.810	1.62
$MgCl_2 \cdot 6H_2O$	0.49	0.0996	0.1992	0.498	0.996
Na lactate	3.30	0.616	1.232	3.08	6.16
(60% syrup)		(280.25 μl)	(560.25 μl)	(1,401.25 μl)	(2, 802.5 μl)

Stock D (calcium) 100×; 1 month expiration

Reagent	*mM*	*g/10 ml*	*g/20 ml*	*g/50 ml*
$CaCl_2 \cdot 2H_2O$	1.71	0.252	0.504	1.260

Stock G (glucose) 10×; 3 months expiration

Reagent	*mM*	*g/10 ml*	*g/50 ml*	*g/100 ml*
Glucose	1.50	0.0270	0.135	0.270

Stock HEPES (HEPES) 10×; 3 months expiration

Reagent	*mM*	*g/50 ml*	*g/100 ml*	*g/200 ml*
HEPES, acid	21	2.9795	5.958	11.916
Phenol red (0.5% solution)		(0.69 ml)	0.0069 g(1.38 ml)	(2.76 ml)

Place approximately 400 ml milliQ water in a 1,000 ml beaker with a stir bar. Mix solutions according to the following directions under the hood:

Stock solution	*HEPES (1 l)*
A (base)	100 ml
D ($CaCl_2$)	10 ml
G (glucosc)	100 ml
NEAA	10 ml
EAA	20 ml
HEPES	84 ml

Place beaker on the stir plate. To the solution add:

Chemical	*For 1 l*
$NaHCO_3$	0.336 g
Napyruvate	0.036g
Glutamine	0.146 g
Fraction V BSA	1.0 g
Gentamycin	1,000 μl
Amphotercin (fungizone)	1,000 μl

Let the solution stir gently until BSA dissolves. This may take a while. Bring volume to approximately 900 ml. pH solution to 7.3–7.4. QS to 1 l. Filter, label and store at 2–8°C.

Caution: pour the solution slowly down the side of the volumetric to avoid bubbling.

Essential and non essential amino acids are purchased from ICN (ICN Biochemicals, Aurora, OH);

(a) 1601149 essential amino acids, 50 ×

(b) 1681049 non essential amino acids, 100 ×

Amphotercin (Fungazone; # 15290–018) from Gibco (Rockville, MD) Gentamycin (# G 1397) from Sigma (St. Louis, MO)

NCSU 23

Component	*g/l*	*mM*
NaCl	6.35	108.7
KCl	0.356	4.78
KH_2PO_4	0.162	1.19
$MgSO_4 \cdot 7H_2O$	0.294	1.19
$NaHCO_3$	2.106	25.07
Glutamine	0.146	1.0
Glucose	1.0	5.55
Taurine	0.876	7.00
Hypotaurine	0.545	5.00
$CaCl_2 \cdot 2H_2O$	0.189	1.70
BSA fractionV (Sigma 3311)	4.0	
Phenol Red, 0.5% (Sigma P0290)	1:0 ml	
Penicillin/Streptomycin (Sigma P0781)	10:0 ml	

Note: All chemicals should be of embryo culture quality. Place components 1–9 in an acid-washed or oven-baked 1l volumetric flask and add embryo culture quality water to about one-half the volume of the round base of the flask. Swirl gently to get all of the components into solution.

1. In a separate 50 ml beaker that has been properly cleaned, completely dissolve the $CaCl_2$ $2H_2O$ in 20 ml embryo culture grade water. After components 1–9 are in solution add the $CaCl_2$ $2H_2O$ slowly and drop- wise to the hand-swirled flask (if a white precipitate forms, start over from scratch). Once components 1-10 are in solution, add the BSA to the medium.
2. Allow the BSA to float on top of the medium and slowly dissolve into the solution. Once components 1-11 are in solution, add the phenol red and antibiotics and bring volume to exactly 1 l with embryo culture grade H_2O. Filter-sterilize the medium through a 0:2 μm vacuum filter flask (Nalgene 154–0020).

PPM media system

Purdue Porcine Media for porcine maturation, fertilization and embryo culture.

1. PPM Base (10 × stock, 1 month expiration; start with 50 ml milliQ H_2O, add reagents, QS to 100 ml)

Reagent	*MW*	*Concentration in final final working solution (mM)*	*g/100 ml for 10× stock*
$NaCl_2$	58.44	100	5.8440
KCl	74.55	5.0	0.3728
KH_2PO_4	136.1	0.50	0.0681
$CaCl_2$	111.0	1.70	0.1887
$MgSO_4 \cdot 7H_2O$	246.5	1.19	0.2933
Alanine	89.09	0.50	0.0446
Glycine	75.07	2.0	0.1501
Phenol red	354.4	0.014 (0.0005%)	0.0050

2. 10 × Stock solutions

Stock	*MW*	*Concentration in final working solution (mM)*	*g/10 ml for 10 × stock*	*Expiration*
Bicarbonate ($NaHCO_3$)	84.01	25	0.21	1 week
Glucose	180. 2	2.0	0.0360	1 month
L-Lactate	90.08	6.0	0.0541	1 month
Pyruvate	110.0	0.2	0.0022	1 week
Taurine	125.1	5.0	0.0626	1 month
Hypotaurine	109.1	5.0	0.0546	1 week

3. 100 × Stock solutions

Stock	*MW*	*Concentration in final working solution (mM)*	*g/10 ml for 100 × stock*	*Expiration*
Glutamine (GLN)	146.15	1.0	0.1461	1 week
Cysteamine	77.14	0.5	0.0386	1 week
Cysteine	175.64	0.57	0.10	1 week
Citrate	294.1	0.5	0.1471	1 week

4. PPM Media

Note: All volumes given in the following table are in microliters unless otherwise stated.

Stock	*PPMmat.*	*PPMfert.*	*PPM1*	*PPM2*
MilliQ water	1,750	1,220	1,600	1,303
Base	500	500	500	500
Bicarbonate	500 (25 mM)	880 (44 mM)	500 (25 mM)	500 (25 mM)

Glucose	500 (2 mM)	100 (0.4 mM)	100 (0.4 mM)	1,500 (6 mM)
L-Lactate	500 (6 mM)	500 (6 mM)	500 (6 mM)	167 (2.04 mM)
Pyruvate	25 (0.01 mM)	500 (0.2 mM)	500 (0.2 mM)	250 (0.1 mM)
Glutamine	50 (1 mM)	50 (1 mM)	50 (1 mM)	75 (1.5 mM)
Taurine	500 (5 mM)	700 (7 mM)	700 (7 mM)	500 (5 mM)
Hypotaurine		500	500	
Cysteamine	50			
Cysteine	50			
Citrate	50			
Caffeine, 2.06 mM		0.002 g		
NEAA, 1×	50	50	50	50
EAA, 0.5×	50			50
Vitamins, 1×	50			50
Hyaluronate, 0.5 mg/ml	250			
BSA, 2 mg/ml fert, 4 mg/ml culture		0.010 g fatty acid free	0.020 g pentex	0.020 g pentex
LH, 0.01 U/ml	25			
FSH, 0.01 U/ml	25			
EGF, 50 ng/ml	25			
Insulin/ transferrin/ selenium (ITS), (I=5 pg/ml, T=5 pg/ml, S=5 ng/ml)	50 1×			50
GH, 100 ng/ml				
Total volume	5 ml	5 ml	5 ml	5 ml

Timeline

This detailed protocol, which is used in the Krisher laboratory:

–4 h	Prepare maturation dishes and allow to equilibrate in incubator
0 h	Arrival of ovaries, collection of oocytes and incubation for maturation. Make mTBM fertilization medium working solution and incubate to equilibrate
+24 h	Prepare mTBM fertilization drops and sperm wash medium, or PPMfert medium and drops. Also prepare SOF HEPES and D-PBS
+38 h	Make 45% and 90% Percoll
+40–42 h	Thaw sperm, separate and count. Denude oocytes. Co-incubate sperm and oocytes for 5 h
+42 h	Prepare zygote culture dishes and incubate
+45–47 h	Place fertilized zygotes into culture
+52–54 h	Mount and fix zygotes on slides to check for fertilization, if desired
+189–191 h	Score for cleavage and development (144 h post culture)

Oocyte Collection and In Vitro Maturation (Day 1)

Reagents required

1. SOF HEPES, (HEPES), medium
2. maturation medium (TCM199 or PPMmat.)
3. Sigma mineral oil, embryo-tested

On the morning ovaries are expected, make your working media for the day. If the PPM system is being used, media should be prepared the evening before use to allow sufficient equilibration time. Make sure that 1 l saline is placed in a warm oven. Aliquot 100 ml HEPES medium into a bottle and place it in the dry oven to warm as well. Make the appropriate maturation medium (TCM199 or PPMmat). Sigma embryo-tested mineral oil should be used throughout this protocol. Prepare a Nunc four-well plate by placing 500 μl of the appropriate maturation medium into each well and cover with about 400 μl mineral oil. One well is used for washing. Place the Nunc plate in the 5% CO_2 in air incubator at 39°C to equilibrate, preferably for 4 h. Both maturation and fertilization are carried out at 39°C.

1. Set up for aspiration. When the ovaries arrive, take the temperature of the ovaries and the saline. Pour the ovaries into a strainer and

wash them twice with the warmed saline, then place them in a beaker and fill the beaker with fresh warm saline so that the ovaries are covered. Do this quickly so they do not get cold. Place the beakers on a slide warmer by the aspiration pump.

2. Aspirate follicles ranging in size from 3 to 8 mm in diameter on the ovary. Pierce the surface of the ovary just outside the visible boundary of the follicle. Go into the follicle under the surface of the ovary, and collect the fluid. While aspirating the fluid, use the needle to scrape the follicle walls to ensure the oocyte is recovered. To avoid loss of fluid, keep the bevel of the needle pointed down and away from you. Collect the fluid in 50 ml tubes.
3. All work with oocytes and embryos in this protocol should be performed as quickly as possible. All dishes containing oocytes or embryos should be worked with on slide warmers where possible, and time out of the incubator for all oocytes, embryos and/or dishes should be minimized. Opening of the incubator door should always be minimized, in regard to number of times opened, length of time open, and width of opening. Red light should be used whenever oocytes or embryos are out of the incubator, because natural light wavelengths can be harmful to oocyte and embryo development. Extended exposure to adverse conditions will result in reduced embryo viability or death.
4. Set up dishes to be used in the search for oocytes: 1× Falcon 1007 dish, 2× Falcon 1008 dishes, several grid dishes (number of tubes of follicular fluid +1), a Drummond pipette with tips, and a sterile disposable transfer pipette. Draw 7–8 lines on the bottom of the 1007 dish. Fill the 1007 and 1008 dishes with HEPES medium – you can either pour or pipette. Aspirate, or sweep, the pellet at the bottom of one aspiration tube using the transfer pipette. Pull sediment (cellular debris and oocyte cumulus complexes) off the bottom of the 50 ml tube into the pipette, using a circular motion. Place the sediment in a grid dish and add HEPES medium. Swirl to mix. With a new Drummond tip, search the grid dish for oocytes.

   The magnification should be such that one square of the grid dish fits in the field of view. Perform some oocyte selection at this time. Ultimately, only oocytes completely covered with cumulus cells that are tightly compacted, and with an even cytoplasm (not pycnotic) will be selected. Also pay attention to the size of the oocyte cytoplasm. If the cytoplasm appears smaller than normal, do not select it. Do not select oocytes with expanded cumulus masses, or with no or incomplete cumulus layers. At this time only a brief look should be given each oocyte. Most oocytes will be removed from the grid dish at this time unless they are obviously poor (such as denuded or expanded). Use the Drummond pipette to pick the oocytes out of the grid dish and move them into the 1007 dish. Search the entire grid dish for oocytes. After the first search, swirl the dish again and search again. Repeat this procedure for each tube. Do a second sweep on all the tubes combined (all second sweeps in one grid dish) when finished with all the first sweeps.

5. When all the oocytes have been collected in the 1007 dish, change the Drummond tip (sterilize the stylet of the pipette with alcohol). Increase the magnification and examine each oocyte line by line in the 1007 dish for the selection criteria described above. Pick up selected oocytes that meet the criteria and place them into the first 1008 dish. When all oocytes have been examined and either selected or rejected, wash the selected oocytes through the remaining 1008 dish. If oocytes that should not be selected become apparent during the washes, they should be discarded at this time.
6. Remove the Nunc four-well dish with maturation medium from the incubator. Place oocytes from the final 1008 wash dish into the wash well, swirl and then distribute to the culture wells, 50 oocytes per 500 μl Nunc well. Place the maturation wells back in the incubator. Oocytes are matured in this medium for 40–42 h in 6% CO_2 in air at 39°C.
7. On this day be sure to record in your notebook:
   - when the ovaries arrived
   - temperature of ovaries on arrival
   - temperature of saline
   - when aspiration began and ended
   - number of ovaries you aspirated
   - when the oocytes went into maturation medium
   - how many oocytes were recovered
   - maturation treatments/medium used
8. Also on this day make fertilization medium working solution and place in the incubator to equilibrate if using the mTBM fertilization medium. Do this in the afternoon.

In vitro maturation (day 2)

Reagents required

- Fertilization medium (mTBM or PPMfert)
- Sperm wash medium
- Percoll
- SOF HEPES, (HEPES)
- D-PBS

1. Oocytes remain in the maturation wells today.
2. In the afternoon, make fertilization drops if using mTBM. Drops should contain 50 μl medium; 20 oocytes will be fertilized per drop. Also make a wash dish with 3 $\times$ 250 μl drops. When making drops, place one-half the volume of the drop in the Falcon 1007 dish, cover with 10 ml mineral oil, then add the remaining drop volume. Place in the incubator (5% CO_2 in air) to equilibrate. In the PPM system, medium and drops are made on this day.
3. Also in the afternoon, make 50 ml sperm wash working solution in a bottle and place in a warm oven if using mTBM. Also prepare and warm 10 ml each SOF HEPES and D-PBS.

In Vitro Fertilization

Reagents required

- mTBM or PPMfert
- 90 and 45% Percoll
- D-PBS sperm wash working solution – D-PBS
- SOF HEPES, (HEPES)

1. In the morning of the day of fertilization, make sure the slide warmers and water bath are turned on. Make 45% (2 ml; 1 ml 90% +1 ml D-PBS with no BSA) and 90% Percoll (1.5 ml) solutions and place in a warm oven. Place the centrifuge buckets in a warm oven as well.
2. The first task is to denude the oocytes of cumulus mass cells. If you are experienced, you can do this during the first Percoll spin, but it must be accomplished in less than 20 min. If you are relatively inexperienced, denude the oocytes first then prepare the sperm. The oocytes should be fertilized 40–42 h post maturation. There are two methods for denuding the oocytes. For most uses, vortexing is the easiest. For nuclear transfer, use the Pipetman. In this case, minimize the exposure of oocytes to hyaluronidase as much as possible.

(a) *Vortexing*. Place 100 μl warmed HEPES into a 1.5 ml microfuge tube. Add 1 μl hyaluronidase solution. Get out 2 × 1008 dishes, fill one with HEPES. Get out the maturation wells, remove the oocytes from the wells using the Drummond and place them in the microfuge tube. Vortex the tube for 3 min. Rinse the tube with HEPES and place the contents in the empty 1008 dish. Repeat twice more. The denuded oocytes will now be in the 1008 dish.

(b) *Pipetting*. Prepare Falcon 3037 dishes by adding 4 ml HEPES to the outer moat, and 1 ml to the inner well. Add 10 μl hyaluronidase solution to the inner well. Take the maturation dishes out of the incubator. Using a cleaned Drummond, remove the oocytes from the maturation drops and transfer them into the inner well. Do only as many as you can quickly process at a time. After placing them into the hyaluronidase well, use a Pipetman set to 100–200 μl and quickly draw the oocytes in and out several times. Once a few oocytes are completely denuded, move them out of the hyaluronidase solution into the HEPES in the moat with the Drummond. Go back and denude a few more with the Pipetman. Repeat this process until all the oocytes in that group are denuded and in the moat. Using the Drummond, remove the group from the moat into a new 1008 dish with HEPES medium. Repeat until all oocytes are denuded.

3. Swirl the 1008 dish with the newly denuded oocytes to rinse well. All hyaluronidase must be rinsed away. After swirling, move the oocytes into the clean HEPES in the second 1008 dish in as little medium as possible. Swirl again. Collect into a group.
4. Move the oocytes into the fertilization medium wash drops. Wash them vigorously through all three wash drops by pulling oocytes and medium up and down rapidly in the Drummond. When all the oocytes are in the final fertilization wash drop, get the previously prepared fertilization drops out of the incubator. From the wash dish, move the oocytes into the fertilization drops with as little medium as possible (20 oocytes per drop).
5. Once the oocytes are denuded and in the fertilization drops, you are ready to begin preparing the sperm. Make a Percoll gradient by gently layering 1.5 ml 45% Percoll on top of the 1.5 ml 90% Percoll in the existing 15 ml blue cap centrifuge tube. Frozen sperm: to thaw the sperm, drop two frozen pellets into 2 ml

warmed HEPES in a small snap cap tube, mix gently once thawed. Layer this 2 ml gently onto the Percoll gradient. Fresh/chilled sperm: Remove 1 ml extended chilled semen from the large 50 ml blue capped tube in the chiller (mix before removing) and warm in a small snap cap tube. Place 500 μl fresh/chilled semen onto the Percoll gradient. Spin the Percoll for 20 min at 700 g (2,100 rpm). Remove the supernatant down to the pellet. Add 5 ml sperm wash medium (mTBM system) or D-PBS (PPM system) to the pellet and flick it gently with your finger to mix the pellet well. Spin for 5 min at 700 g. Again, remove the supernatant down to the pellet, and repeat the rinse. After the final spin, add 100 μl fertilization medium to the pellet and mix gently by hand.

6. Prepare the dilution tubes for sperm counting. Fill one 1.5 ml microfuge tube with 900 μl water and label 1,000 ×, and one with 990 μl water and label 100 ×. Add 10 μl sperm solution to the 100 × tube, mix well. Take 100 μl of this solution and add it to the 1,000 × tube. Mix well. Place the sperm solution, as well as the remaining fertilization medium, in the incubator for 1 h.
7. Count the sperm and dilute. Place 10 μl 1,000 × dilution on each side of the haemocytometer. Count the four large grid boxes on each side of the haemocytometer (a total of eight boxes). Divide the total sperm counted by eight. This is the average count per square, or x. Multiply by 10 (each square of the haemocytometer has a volume of 0.1 mm^3) $=10 \times$ sperm/μl. Multiply by 1,000 to account for the dilution factor, and multiply by 1,000 again to get sperm/ml. Thus, average count × 107 is sperm/ml. The final sperm concentration in the fertilization drop should be 500,000 sperm/ml. Thus, we need to add 50,000 sperm in 50 μl to give a total of 50,000 sperm in the 100 μl drop. 50,000 sperm in 50 μl = 1 million sperm/ml. This is the correct sperm dilution. To calculate how much of the sperm pellet and how much of the fertilization medium to mix to make a 1 million sperm/ml suspension, use the following calculation:

$$\frac{\text{Average count} \times 10^7}{1{,}000\ \mu\text{l}} = \frac{1 \times 10^6}{x\ \mu\text{l}}$$

Solve for x. This is the amount of the sperm pellet to add. Subtract this number from 1,000 to get the amount of fert medium to add. Examples:

(a) If your total count of eight boxes was 12 sperm: 12 ÷ 8 = 1.5, so there are 1.5×10^7 sperm/ml in the sperm pellet tube.

$$\frac{1.5\times10^{7}\ \text{sperm / ml}}{1{,}000\ \mu\text{l}}=\frac{1\times10^{6}\ \text{sperm / ml}}{x\ \mu\text{l}} \qquad ...(1)$$

x = 66.7 μl to make the final sperm suspension, add 66.7 μl of the sperm pellet to 933.3 μl fert medium (1,000–66.7) in a microfuge tube.

(b) If the total count of eight boxes was 168: 168 ÷ 8 = 21

$$\frac{2.1\times10^{7}\ \text{sperm / ml}}{1{,}000\ \mu\text{l}}=\frac{1\times10^{6}\ \text{sperm / ml}}{x\ \mu\text{l}} \qquad ...(2)$$

x = 4.8 μl to make the final sperm suspension, add 4.8 μl of the sperm pellet to 995.2 μl fert medium (1,000–4.8) in a microfuge tube.

In the calculation, if you need to inseminate with a final sperm concentration other than 500,000/ml, substitute 1×10^6 sperm/ml in the equation for the following:

250,000, use 0.5×10^6

500,000, use 1×10^6

1 million, use 2×10^6

2 million, use 4×10^6

8. Remove the fertilization drops containing oocytes from the incubator. Place them on the slide warmer. Using a Pipetman, add 50 μl of the sperm dilution. Check to be sure that you have added sperm to all drops containing oocytes and put the dishes back into the incubator. Clean up the area. Record in your notebook the time the oocytes were moved to fertilization drops, the counts, the dilution made, and the time the sperm was added to the oocytes. Co-incubate oocytes and sperm for 5 h.

In Vitro Culture

Reagents required

- NCSU23 or PPMI [followed by PPM2 at 72 hpi (hours post insemination)]

1. The presumptive zygotes should be placed into culture 5 hpi. This is the same day as fertilization. Embryos are cultured at 39°C in 6% CO_2 and 10% O_2, balanced with N_2. On the day of fertilization and culture, you should make the appropriate culture medium (NCSU23 or PPM 1) immediately after fertilization. Make drops (25 μl + 10 ml oil +25 μl) in 1007 dishes as well as three 250 μl drops (125 μl + oil +125 μl) in a 1007 dish for washing. Place in the incubator to equilibrate. The drops should equilibrate at least 3 h before adding the zygotes.

2. Remove the fertilization and the culture medium wash dish from the culture incubator. Wash the fertilized zygotes well through all three wash drops of the culture medium. (If you are mounting embryos on a slide to check for fertilization, place the zygotes to be mounted in the wash drops back into the incubator. At 12 hpi, mount them on a slide.)
3. Remove the culture drops from the incubator. Pick up ten embryos in as little medium as possible and place into the final culture drop. Place the culture dish back into the incubator. Record the culture medium used, and the time the zygotes were placed into the culture drops.
4. If NCSU23 is used, nothing else is done until day 6. If PPM1/2 is used, embryos are moved from PPM1 to PPM2 at 72 hpi. On day 3 (72 hpi), make PPM2 culture medium. Make culture drops in the morning (25 μl + oil) and allow to equilibrate for at least 3 h. Again, make wash drops in the culture plate as above. At 72 hpi, move the embryos quickly from the original culture drops to the wash drops, wash through three wash drops and distribute ten per 50 μl culture drop. Embryos must be washed thoroughly at this step. Move them in as little of the original medium as possible at each step. Place the new culture drops back into the incubator. Record the date and time when the embryos were moved. NCSU23 allows for continuous culture without intervention or changing of medium. PPM1/2 media are designed to be changed during the culture period. Since NCSU23 does as well or better for most applications, its ease of use argues for its inclusion in transgenic protocols with pigs.
5. At 144 hpi (day 6) post insemination, remove the embryos from the incubator and score each embryo for cleavage and development.

Protocols for In Vivo Production of Pig Embryos

Timeline

-0 h	Receipt of gilts. PMSG dosage (4:00 pm)
+72 h	hCG dosage (4:00 pm)
+114 h	First natural mating of gilts (10:00 am)
+119 h	Second natural mating of gilts (3:00 pm)
+121 h	Withdraw food supply from gilts prior to surgery (5:00 pm)
+138–143 h	Surgery for recovery of embryos (10:00 am–3:00 pm)
+139–141 h	Microinjection of embryos (11:00 am–4:00 pm)
+143–145 h	Transfer of microinjected embryos (3:00–5:00 pm)

Synchronization and Superovulation of Embryo Donors

Sufficient embryo donors and recipients are required to efficiently produce transgenic pigs. In our hands, a minimum of five prepuberal gilts (young female pigs) are required to provide sufficient embryos on average to allow for one successful embryo transfer. Gilts (150-160 days of age) were shipped to our farm on the day superovulation was to begin. Shipping stress may enhance the success of superovulation. Pregnant mare's serum gonadotrophin (PMSG, 1,500 IU) was injected by intramuscular injection (im) at 4:00 pm on the day of arrival. Human chorionic gonadotrophin (hCG, 500 IU, im) was given 72 h after the PMSG injection. In the United States these drugs are not approved for general use in pigs and must be cleared through Federal and State authorities. Special permission will be required. The gilts were then mated by natural service or artificial insemination at 42 and 47 h after the hCG injection. The synchronization of gilts is an advantage in this procedure since the gilts are bred by artificial insemination on a timed basis, irrespective of oestrus behavior. Oestrus is the period during which the female is receptive to mating by the male. When properly stimulated, she assumes a characteristic "*standing oestrus*" pose indicating receptivity. Oestrus in the pig lasts for 3 days. Natural mating may result in ovulation occurring during a fairly broad time frame during oestrus. Superovulation with gonadotrophins in prepubertal females "sets" the system so that we can better predict the time of ovulation. Two inseminations are given to be sure of fertilization. Because oestrous behavior is variable, inseminations are given regardless of behavior. Exceptionally good results have been obtained with this system of reproductive management. Our experience indicates that virtually every donor ovulates using this protocol and will produce fertilized embryos if inseminated. Without synchronization, one would not know when to breed or when ovulation was occurring during the 3 day oestrous period. Synchronization also allows a greater number of embryo donors to be handled on the same day, which may be important for obtaining sufficient embryos for transfer. Surgical collection should start on the morning after insemination. Most of the embryo donors can be expected to have more than 20 embryos. Thus, a group of five donors should yield on average 100 embryos for microinjection. Experiments should be avoided when the ambient temperature is very high, due to the effects of high temperature on fertility. These effects become evident in males, which exhibit a pronounced sterility; and also in females, which undergo a behavioral depression.

Embryo Recovery

Embryo recovery in the pig requires surgery and may be intimidating to most laboratories. If this is the case, collaboration with laboratory animal experts may be warranted. The strategy to be used is to enter the body cavity, exteriorize the oviducts, and flush them with embryo culture medium. Details on the anaesthesia and the surgery are best described by surgical experts (Swindle 1998) as a number of different protocols are possible.

Reagents required

- NCSU23

Preparation for surgery

1. Pigs are fasted from solid food for at least 6–8 h
2. When going into surgery, the pig is draped to prevent hypothermia
3. Monitoring may be accomplished by noting respiration and using a pulse oximeter
4. An injectable or inhalation anaesthesia may be used
5. Example anaesthesia protocol,

Induction	
Ketamine	33 mg/kg im
Acepromazine	1.1 mg/kg im
Atropine	0.05 mg/kg im
Maintenance	
Isofluorane	1.5%–2% in oxygen or 0.5%–1.5% in nitrous oxide; oxygen 2:1

6. One person (the anesthesiologist) must monitor the vital signs of the patient during the surgery. The time required for surgery must be minimized; no more that 30 min from the time of induction of anaesthesia to removal from isofluorane is a good goal to try to achieve.

Surgical technique for skin opening and closure

These techniques are discussed in Swindle's books. The choice of instruments is important, as are the suture and needles. Our own suture methods have evolved over time. The reason for this is that the abdominal incision in a large pig is subject to a lot of abdominal pressure, and scratching may damage the suture line on the skin. On the internal suture line of peritoneum and linea alba taken up together, we insert the needle about 12.5 mm on each side of the incision using synthetic suture, thus turning the edges of the suture line slightly up. In addition, each stitch is "locked" by turning the suture loop and pulling the needle through it. Consequently, there is little chance that any of these pigs will ever develop a hernia. The skin incision could also be a problem. If scratched, the suture may dehisce. We use a "box" stitch with cat gut that is absorbable and thus does not have to be removed later. After appropriate withdrawal times, embryo donors went on to slaughter and embryo recipients were held for anticipation of pregnancy and parturition about 4 months later.

Embryo collection

Our protocol was originally developed at North Carolina State University in the 1960s by L. C. Ulberg – a pioneer in embryo transfer research.

Blunt dissection (using only fingers) is used through the substantial fat layer found between the skin and the connective tissue overlying the abdominal cavity. A ~ 5–7:5 cm incision is made in the linea alba (midventral connective tissue between abdominal muscles) to reveal the abdominal region. The abdominal cavity is entered by "poking" with a finger to pierce the peritoneum and then enlarging the hole to the size of the incision in the linea alba. One reproductive tract is exteriorized at a time, and the oviducts flushed with sterile medium. After both sides have been flushed, the reproductive tracts are carefully returned to the abdominal cavity and the incisions closed immediately unless the animal is to be held for use as an embryo recipient.

For recovery of one cell embryos, a bent glass cannula (sized to fit the embryo donors being used – a range should be available when first starting), flared at one end, is placed in the upper end of the oviduct, the infundibulum, which is a large membraneous structure that enshrouds the ovary. The cannula can be carefully clamped, but we have found much better results if a surgical assistant holds the cannula in place between thumb and forefinger and directs the end of the cannula to the collection dish. The surgeon now uses syringe and blunted needle (18 g) to cannulate the uterine tubule junction (UTJ) and complete a retrograde flush of the oviduct using 15–20 ml embryo culture medium (NCSU-23). A team of at least three people are required for the surgical activity (surgeon and assistant + anesthesiologist). This team of three continues to isolate embryos in the surgery while a second team of at least two people will handle and microinject the embryos in a separate room very close to the surgery. As soon as embryos are obtained, they are taken for processing and microinjection. Close coordination of recovery, microinjection and transfer became a key goal of the teamwork approach.

PRODUCTION OF TRANSGENIC PIGS

Centrifugation and Microinjection of Embryos

Pig embryos are sensitive to low temperature, so room temperature (assumed to be 25°C) is kept a few degrees higher if possible (25–38°C). Even room temperature is a risk to pig embryos. Warming trays and in cubators are to ensure that the embryos never experience temperature below 38°C except for short periods of time - even the microfuge is placed inside an incubator, although the incubator must be monitored for heat build up. During microinjection, a heated stage is used to maintain embryo viability. Water-jacketed tissue-culture incubators are used. Cheaper, air-jacketed, thermal incubators must never be used because the temperature may reach levels higher than desired. Temperature calibration of incubators and other such devices must be determined and verified by the average of three calibrated thermometers. Never autoclave anything that will come into contact with embryos because of steam cleaning residues - instead use high dry heat (glassware), boiling water (plastic tubing) and filter (media) sterilization.

Handling of embryos is kept to a minimum and must always be carried out in an efficient manner. NCSU-23 is used at all times and must be gassed with 5% CO_2. Whatever medium is used, switching to different media during the course of the experiment is discouraged, as is the use of oil overlays (except during microinjection and fertilization). Embryos are recovered from the oviductal flush in gridded plastic plates that can easily hold 15–25 ml fluid that allow for the dispersal of debris. The embryos have a very dark, dense cytoplasm and are easily visible in the plate of flushing medium. Embryos are collected using a mouth-controlled Pasteur pipette (pulled, and broken or cut to a working size tip). Embryos are washed a number of times and quickly placed in the incubator prior to centrifugation and microinjection.

Centrifugation allows visualization of the pronuclei. Embryos are placed in a standard microcentrifuge tube and centrifuged for a few minutes. Each laboratory will have to titrate this method to find the time that works best for visualizing the pronuclei. Consult the paper of for more details on the technique, which is surprisingly easy to master.

Standard microinjection procedures using a heated stage can be used in the pig once the pronuclei are visible after centrifugation.

While microinjection procedures may be standard, we have found two problems that may occur and which individual laboratories may have to grapple with, at least at some level. These are: making and filling the injection pipette, and achieving and maintaining adequate flow for microinjection. We have found that injection pipettes with internal capillaries fill best and whereas these used to be custom-made in the lab, they can now be purchased. Flow can be a problem because injection pipettes may have such a small opening that sufficient pressure cannot be generated to cause fluid to flow out. Hydrofluoric acid (HF) can be used to open the injection pipette once the pipette is loaded and attached to the microinjection setup.

Note: HF is a potentially harmful chemical. Consult with your Safety Office regarding handling, use and disposal.

Procedure for opening the tip of the microinjection pipette

A standard, plastic culture dish, such as a Falcon 3002, is used to hold the HF microdroplets. First, a 5 μl drop of HF is placed in the dish. Smaller droplets are made around the first drop. These droplets, in turn, are used to open the tip of the needle. Embryo culture quality mineral oil is used to overlay the HF droplets. The tip of the DNA-loaded needle is lowered into the oil and placed near one of the smaller droplets. The pressure to the injecting needle is then increased while the tip of the needle is directed into the HF droplet. Once flow is observed, the tip of the needle is moved out of the HF droplet and a small pool of DNA buffer is allowed to form around the tip of the needle as the flow dynamics of the needle are assessed by the operator. It may be necessary to repeat this procedure to get adequate flow.

This method has worked very well for us and was used in the production of our rhodopsin transgenic pigs. In our experience, survival after microinjection can be very high.

Embryo Recipient Selection and Embryo Transfer

Select small pigs and pigs with badly conformed legs for the first set of surgeries. These pigs will not be used as recipients. The best pigs are saved for the last surgeries and the best one or two of these (normal ovarian morphology, ovulation sites and no cysts), normal embryo number (10–25) and morphology (one-cell) are chosen as recipients for the microinjected embryos.

A total of 40–60 microinjected embryos are transferred to each recipient female. Either 20–30 can be transferred to each side or all embryos can be transferred to one side because the embryos will be transported and spaced evenly throughout both uterine horns. Survival at microinjection is not assessed. Instead, all microinjected embryos are speedily transferred to a recipient female. The embryos are carefully loaded into a 10 μl micropipette attached to a positive displacement micropipette by flexible tubing. The positive displacement pipette is an advantage because maximum control over flow is achieved and accidental problems such as temperature-induced volume changes are minimized. Using a dissecting microscope, load the micropipette. This can be a challenge because it must be held perpendicular to the bottom of the dish and the embryos and air bubbles must be loaded within the displacement of the micropipette. A hole is made in the upper end of the oviduct (precise location is important) with a blunt needle, and the embryos carefully deposited in the oviduct in a minimal volume of medium, by first inserting the micropipette using the naked eye. Air bubbles in the capillary tube serve as convenient markers indicating when the embryos have entered the oviduct. Many laboratories use plastic tubing attached to a 1 ml syringe to instill the embryos directly into the upper end of the oviducts. Some possible problems include losing embryos (and perhaps not realizing it – this is especially a problem for the syringe method) and not placing the embryos in the proper location (not in the upper end of the oviduct, for instance). Generally, however, embryo transfer in the pig is routine and has a very high success rate.

Methods for Animal Identification

As with other transgenic animals, identification systems must be accurate and not likely to be lost or confused during the animal's lifetime. Founder animals must be screened with Southern blots that demonstrate unique flanking regions. This is absolutely required. Subsequently, PCR screens can be used and reconfirmed with Southern blots if required. When the pig is young, the tail is normally docked. This is the tissue used for DNA analysis. In pigs, tattoos are possible but are often difficult to read due to skin pigmentation and changes in size with growth. Ear notches and ear tags are used to identify pigs. In addition, cage cards with appropriate information are prominently displayed.

9

Transgenic Birds

The generation of transgenic birds using lentiviral vectors is an efficient procedure that is relatively simple compared to the production of transgenic mice and other mammals. Most tools and reagents required are available in a typical molecular biology laboratory, and the procedure can be performed on a laboratory bench without special concerns for sterility. The method for avian transgenesis described here is similar to previous methods used to produce transgenic chickens by the microinjection of recombinant oncoretroviruses into the early embryo of freshly laid eggs. However, lentiviral transgenesis has a number of important advantages over previous methods. The primary advantage of using lentiviral vectors is that they are not subject to the silencing that oncoretroviral-based vectors undergo in the developing embryo. Previous studies of transgenic chickens and quails produced with oncoretroviral vectors reported low or undetectable levels of transgene expression. In contrast, we and others have demonstrated that lentiviral vectors allow for high levels of transgene expression in quails and chickens. Additionally, we have shown that lentiviral vectors allow for tissue-specific expression in transgenic birds. Transgenesis using lentiviruses has been shown to be a versatile and powerful genetic tool in mice. In this chapter we describe the application of this tool to birds. Although this system has only been tested in chickens and quails, we anticipate that lentiviral transgenesis will be possible in a wide variety of avian species.

Overview of the Strategy

In birds, after fertilization of the oocyte by the sperm has occurred, the embryo starts developing inside the female's reproductive tract until the egg is laid a few hours later. During the migration of the fertilized embryo through the reproductive tract, two key processes occur simultaneously. First, the cells in the embryo proliferate rapidly in such a way that by the time the egg is laid (3–5 days postfertilization) the embryo will consists of 20,000–50,000 cells (depending on the species). Second, during migration the egg will acquire a calcerous shell. Therefore, once the embryo has completed its intrauterine migration, the female will lay a single embryo consisting of tens of thousand of cells, which is surrounded by an opaque shell. These special characteristics of avian development pose some obstacles to the generation of transgenic birds. First, the embryo cannot be easily observed with a microscope, because the shell prevents its visualization. Second, because the embryo consists of some 20,000–40,000 cells it will not be possible to deliver transgenes to 100% of the embryonic cells. Accordingly, the strategy for transgenesis in birds is based on the delivery of transgenes to a percentage of the cells of the founder embryo. When this embryo develops, it will become a mosaic animal (F_0), in which a percentage of cells will contain the transgene. If some of the transgene-carrying cells in the F_0 mosaic founder differentiate into sperm or oocytes, then when these mosaic founder animals breed they will pass the transgene to a percentage of their progeny (F_1), which will become transgenic birds carrying a copy of the transgene in all cells of the body.

Design of Lentiviral Vectors for Transgene Expression

A general introduction to the design and construction of lentiviral vectors is given elsewhere in this book, Generation of Transgenic Animals Using Lentiviral Vectors. However, there are some specific considerations for the design of vectors used to make transgenic birds.

Promoters

The appropriate choice of cis-regulatory elements used to drive trans- gene expression is critical to the successful generation of useful trans- genic animals. A variety of enhancer/promoter combinations are available to drive transgene expression ubiquitously, or in specific tissues, or at different times during development. However, most well characterized promoters have been studied only in mice or other mammals. Some promoter/enhancer combinations can have quite different transcriptional activity in mice than in birds, which can lead to changes in tissue specificity or overall expression level from species to species. These differences in gene expression can often be difficult to predict, especially when the promoter is a viral sequence that shares no homology with regulatory elements in the avian genome, such as the immediate early promoter from the human *cytomegalovirus* (CMV). In mice, the CMV promoter is commonly used to produce animals with strong transgene expression in most tissues. In contrast, transgenic chickens made to carry the CMV promoter driving the *green fluorescent protein* (GFP) exhibited transgene expression primarily in the pancreas and skin, and very weak expression in other tissues. In addition, expression was not reported in some cell types, notably neurons, which exhibit strong transgene expression from the CMV promoter in mice. Another promoter used to drive constitutive transgene expression in mice, the promoter from the human ubiquitin-C gene, produces only low levels of transgene expression in quail. We have found two promoter/enhancer combinations that produce experimentally useful patterns of gene expression in transgenic quail. Using vectors carrying the human synapsin gene I promoter we have produced a line of transgenic quail with neuron-specific expression of GFP. Additionally, we found that the combination of the CMV enhancer and the chicken β-actin promoter produces ubiquitous expression in quail.

Before using a promoter/enhancer combination that has not been well characterized in birds, transcriptional activity should be tested either in cultured cells from that species, or by in ovo injection. Additionally, the transcriptional activity of a promoter may differ from one avian species to another. For instance, we have found that the CMV/β-actin promoter leads to high expression in quail, but very weak expression in zebra finches. Before the generation of transgenics in a novel species, candidate promoters should be tested to determine their activity in that species.

A second important consideration when choosing a promoter/enhancer combination is the possibility of side effects due to high levels of expression from ubiquitous promoters. Some constitutive promoters can overburden the normal transcriptional machinery of the cell, re-directing resources away from genes necessary for cell growth and towards the transgene. This slows cell proliferation, which puts infected cells at a selective disadvantage when compared to the naive, non-infected cells of the embryo, and lowers the germline transmission frequency of adult mosaics. We have observed this problem when generating transgenic quail that ubiquitously express GFP. When mosaic founder parent birds were generated with a lentiviral vector carrying the chicken β-actin promoter and CMV enhancer driving GFP, we found that only one out often founder quail produced transgenic offspring, and germline transmission frequency in those birds was low (<5% of progeny were transgenic). Somatic mosaicism in adult founders was also low (<1% of cells expressed GFP). In contrast, we generated transgenic quails in which GFP was driven by a neuron-specific promoter (human synapsin I), which showed very high levels of germline transmission. Germline transmission frequency in transgenic quail showing neuron-specific expression was between 5% and 33%, and five out of six mosaic quail produced transgenic offspring. Additionally somatic mosaicism in the neuron-specific transgenics was greater, (1–10% of neurons in these animals expressed GFP), than that of quail generated with the chicken β-actin/CMV vector (less than 1% of cells expressed GFP in the mosaic founders). Therefore, special care should be used when choosing promoters that may express in the germline of the developing bird, since the additional demands made on the cell's transcriptional machinery can impede transgenesis. Any manipulation that decreases the growth rate of infected germ cells, may ultimately lower the germline transmission rate of mosaic founders.

Transgenes

Up to 10 kb kb exogenous DNA, including cis-acting regulatory elements and protein-coding or other transcribed sequences, can be packaged between the flanking long terminal repeats of the lentiviral vector. Currently, only the protein markers GFP and beta-galactosidase, have been expressed in transgenic birds generated with lentiviral vectors. However, the range of possible transgenes is quite extensive, and limited only by the space constraints of the vector. Three general types of transgene are available for use with the lentiviral system. (1) Genes of interest can be ectopically expressed in the whole animal or selected tissues, based on the choice of promoter as described above. These might be endogenous genes, overexpressed to examine the effects of dosage on their normal protein function. Alternatively, exogenous genes that code for visible markers or biopharmaceuticals may be expressed. (2) Dominant negative constructs can be delivered that interfere with the function of endogenous genes. (3) Non-coding RNAs, in particular short interfering RNAs (siRNAs), can also be introduced using lentiviral vectors. siRNAs have been shown to be effective in silencing endogenous genes in transgenic mice generated using lentiviral vectors. Importantly, the mouse U6 promoter, which is required to properly transcribe siRNA, has been shown to work effectively in birds. These strategies make lentiviruses useful vectors for genetic manipulation in birds.

Production of Transgenic Birds

Egg Preparation

Fertile eggs from many domestic species including quail, chicken, ducks and turkey are available by mail from farms or other breeders. Since bird embryos will start to develop when kept at room temperature, it is best to select a vendor that can guarantee freshly laid eggs and that can ship overnight. Vendors that specialize in avian research are preferable. We obtain quail eggs from CBT Farms. Orders are typically 100–200 eggs, which are shipped by express courier. If it is not convenient to inject eggs the day they arrive, eggs can be stored for up to 1 week at 15°C in a cold room or refrigerator. When storing eggs for any length of time, we place eggs in a dedicated refrigerator and orient eggs so that the blunt end of the egg faces upward.

Once the eggs arrive in the laboratory, the crates are unpacked and the eggs placed in racks and oriented so that the long axis of the egg is parallel to the ground. Keeping the eggs in this position allows the embryo to settle to the top of the egg so that it will be accessible in the window that will be created later for virus delivery. The eggs are left in racks at room temperature for 1 h, after which time we find that the majority of embryos lie just below the highest point of the shell. We mark this point with a felt tip pen to identify the presumptive location of the embryo.

For the windowing procedure, eggs are transferred to individual soft foam cradles. Using a hand rotary tool with a small bit, a circle with a 4 mm radius is drilled in the shell around the mark indicating the top of the egg. The window should be made shallow to avoid damaging the shell membrane. We have used both electric hand drills and air-powered dental drills to cut the window. Shell chips and dust can accumulate during the windowing. To eliminate this shell dust, dental drills can be purchased with a second channel that expels air at the head of the drill. This air stream is useful for blowing away the shell chips and dust that accumulate during drilling. If shell chips and dust remain after the cutting process, these should be wiped away with a Kimwipe moistened with 70% ethanol.

After the circular cut is made, the remaining shell fragments are removed with sterilized forceps to expose the shell membrane. Before removing the shell membrane, a drop of sterile *phosphate buffered saline* (PBS) large enough to cover the exposed shell membrane is added over the window. It has been shown that addition of PBS before removal of the shell membrane significantly increases hatchability.

The shell membrane is then removed with forceps, taking care not to disrupt the vitelline membrane that surrounds the embryo and yolk.

Injection for the Production of Mosaic Founders (F_0)

Once the shell membrane is removed, the embryo can be observed by the unaided eye. However, for precise targeting of the embryo we place the egg in a soft cradle under a dissecting microscope with 16X magnification.

Microinjection needles are fabricated from borosilicate glass capillary tubes pulled using a Flaming/Brown micropipette puller, model P-97, using the following parameter settings:

Heat = Ramp + 15
Pull = 30
Vel = 120
Time = 200
Pressure = 200

A ceramic tile (Sutter) is used to score and break the pulled glass give a blunt tip with a 20 μm outer diameter. Once cut, the microinjection needle is inserted into the pipette holder of a CellTram hydraulic injector and front-loaded with concentrated viral solution slowly (roughly 200 nl/s). To be able to visualize the viral solution as it is injected, we add the dye Phenol Red (final concentration 5%) before loading the viral solution into the pipette. We typically load 10–15 μl viral solution, mixed with Phenol Red, into a microinjection needle. A fully loaded needle should allow up to five egg injections.

High titer viral stocks are critical for the production of transgenic birds. We have successfully used viral stocks with titers of 10^6 to 10^7 infectious units per microliter (IU/μl) when titered on 293 cells. Using viral stocks of 10^5 IU/μl or lower will result in very low rates of germline transmission frequencies in mosaic birds. Previous studies using unconcentrated retroviral vectors (10^4 IU=μl) to produce transgenic birds have reported low germline transmission frequencies (<1%) in mosaic founders. In addition to using high titer vector stocks, it is important to minimize the time viruses spend in the injection needle, especially under halogen illumination, since vector particles degrade more rapidly at room temperature. To slow this degradation we keep the thawed viral aliquots on ice before loading into the microinjection needle.

Under a dissecting microscope, the microinjection needle is positioned above the center of the embryo using a micromanipulator.

The needle tip is then advanced to penetrate the embryo, at an angle of approximately 45°. A Piezo Drill attached to the microinjection needle can be used to help the needle tip rupture the vitelline membrane and penetrate the embryo. After the embryo has been penetrated, 3 μl vector solution is slowly injected into the subgerminal cavity, below the embryo. An injection is considered successful if the viral solution is observed spreading horizontally in a circle below the embryo and if the perimeter of the viral solution reaches the borders of the area opaca. In our hands more than 90% of injections are successful according to these criteria. Eggs with unsuccessful injections are discarded. For quails or chickens, we routinely inject 60–80 eggs per day. Assuming a hatching rate of 5–10%, this number of injected eggs will provide a sufficient number of founder animals for breeding.

Immediately after a successful injection, eggs are sealed in order to prevent microbial contamination and fluid loss during incubation. To seal the eggshell, a round glass cover slip is placed over the shell window and is sealed to the egg with a biocompatible silicone elastomer (Kwik-Cast WPI). Eggs are placed blunt end up, in a forced air incubator (Brinsea) with a temperature of 38°C and a relative humidity of 45% until hatching roughly 18 days later. The method of egg turning is an important factor to consider when choosing an incubator. Artificial incubator models that keep each egg (or eggs) in a single plastic cradle and change the orientation of the cradle, such as Brinsea and Alpha Genesis, are preferable to incubators that roll the eggs, such as Grumbach.

This simple method of sealing and incubating eggs typically yields a 10% hatch rate. Other incubation methods, both in artificial culture systems and in ovo, have been described that increase the hatching rate up to 30% or 60%. However, since germline transmission rates are high enough in mosaics produced with lentiviral vectors that only a few founders are needed to guarantee transgenic offspring.

Transgenic Offspring

Once mosaic founders have reached sexual maturity (7 weeks after hatching), these animals are bred to wildtype quail. Wildtype quail can be purchased from breeders and are usually inexpensive (<US $10 per adult quail). However, although the price for individual birds is typically low, shipping live birds can be quite expensive (US $300). Therefore, the best strategy is to order additional eggs and let them develop alongside the injected eggs, or alternatively, to breed mosaic founder quail to each other.

Since founder quail will be mosaic in all tissues, including the germ cells, only a percentage of their offspring will be fully transgenic. If the transgene produces a visible marker, such as GFP, the progeny can be screened for the presence of the transgene by phenotype. In general, however, screening is accomplished by either PCR or Southern blot analysis. Genomic DNA is required for both methods and can be easily extracted from the blood of birds. The alar vein of 5-day-old hatchlings is an excellent source of blood. The vein is nicked with a hypodermic needle and 70 μl blood is collected with a heparinized capillary tube. Genomic DNA can be extracted from blood by digesting overnight in proteinase K followed by phenol/chloroform extraction.

Lentiviral vectors integrate stably into the host chromosome and are passed through the germline to subsequent generations. Transgene expression is consistent from generation to generation; therefore positively identified transgenic birds can be used to establish breeding lines.

Husbandry

Husbandry concerns vary from species to species. Our laboratory has experience raising quails (*Coturnix coturnix*) and zebra finches (*Taeniopygia guttata*). Quails are the preferred species for testing injection methods, promoter/enhancers and general troubleshooting because they develop at a rapid rate (becoming sexually mature roughly 50 days after hatching) and because they are easy to house and care for. A colony of 30 breeding quails can be easily established by purchasing ready-to-assemble rack breeder cages, and will only occupy 1.86 m^2 of laboratory space. In contrast, for most laboratories in an academic environment it will be difficult to establish a colony of chickens because their large size will require a special facility for their breeding. Zebra finches require more time to become sexually mature (90 days) and must be raised by foster parents. Tutorials on quail husbandry with an agricultural or research focus are available.

Our quails hatch in the incubator and are immediately transferred to a brooder (Brinsea) maintained at a temperature of 37°C. After 5 days, the hatchlings are transferred to a larger battery cage that has been modified for hatchlings. The floors and sides have been reinforced with tighter mesh wiring (9 mm × 9 mm hole size) and the cage is equipped with an area heater set to produce an average air temperate of 35°C. Quail can also be raised in commercially available brooders, but our design can house both adults and hatchlings on different levels of a single rack of cages. Hatchlings are fed adult food that has been finely ground to a powder in a kitchen blender. Since quail hatchlings can drown in even shallow depths of standing water, we provided drinking water either in low plastic drinking fountains or in shallow tissue culture plates.

POPULATION STRUCTURE AND GENETIC DIVERSITY IN SWAINSON'S HAWKS (*BUTEO SWAINSONI*)

An on-going concern of conservation biology is the maintenance of biodiversity and identification of appropriate biological units for conservation. In order to best preserve existing biodiversity and evolutionary processes in human altered environments, genetic considerations such as population structure and genetic diversity must be incorporated into management strategies. Birds of prey are often typified by large home ranges and low population densities. As human influences continue to alter natural environments raptor populations have become fragmented and have decreased often to the point of endangerment. As populations decline, genetic variability may be lost as populations become subdivided, gene flow is reduced, and inbreeding increases. This pattern is often seen among naturally isolated populations of island endemics, as has been documented in the Galapagos Hawk (*Buteo galapagoensis*) and has also been recorded among raptors in human fragmented landscapes.

Maintenance of genetic diversity among currently widespread raptor species requires determination of population structure and the contemporary genetic diversity within populations. Low genetic differentiation tends to be characteristic of highly mobile species with broad distributions, such as raptors. Observed genetic variation may still be of consequence in conservation efforts, indicating, for example, incipient population divergence or differing selective regimes with ongoing gene flow.

Swainson's Hawks (*Buteo swainsoni*) are designated federally as a Species of Concern in some regions and listed as Threatened by the State of California. The Swainson's Hawk is a large, highly migratory raptor with a breeding distribution that extends across grasslands, open woodlands, and today incorporates many agricultural landscapes of western North America. Swainson's Hawks were historically considered to be one of the most abundant raptor species in western North America, but have declined precipitously in many parts of their range during the 20th century. Declines began during European settlement with many regions experiencing marked declines by 1900. The contemporary range of the Swainson's Hawk includes a contiguous portion of the Great Basin, Great Plains, and southwestern deserts (GBGP) and a geographically disjunct range in central California.

In California there was a precipitous decline in Swainson's Hawk numbers during the 20th century, with the population declining by as much as 90%. Along with a decline in census numbers, the historical range of Swainson's Hawks in California has been much reduced. Populations from coastal southern California and the coastal foothills and plains have been extirpated with populations still existing in portions of the Sacramento-San Joaquin Valleys in central California, the Modoc Plateau in northeastern California, and remnant population in Owen's Valley and the Mojave Desert. Recent threats to the persistence of Swainson's Hawks include pesticide poisonings in wintering ranges resulting in mass mortalities and loss of habitat within the breeding range.

Dispersal between the CV and the GBGP may be limited. Study sites in California have documented high rates of nest site fidelity with mean natal dispersal of less than 10 km and mean adult dispersal of less than 5 km while natal dispersal in excess of 100 km has been observed in Alberta. Behavioral and morphological studies suggest that Swainson's Hawks breeding in the CV might be genetically distinct from those breeding in the GBGP. Banding and telemetry data indicates that Swainson's Hawks from other regions winter in the pampas of Argentina, while the majority of CV Swainson's Hawks winter in western Mexico and Central America. In addition to migratory differences, Swainson's Hawks occurring in California display a much greater frequency of dark, rufous, and intermediate plumaged individuals with local frequencies of approximately 85–90% within the CV compared with less than 40% outside of the state and less than 1% in the GBGP. These dispersal, behavioral and morphological differences between regions along with documented population declines prompted an investigation to determine whether CV Swainson's Hawks are genetically distinct from those in other regions.

This investigation of Swainson' s Hawk genetics had two goals: first, to use a panel of 19 Swainson's Hawk-specific microsatellite loci along with mitochondrial DNA sequence data to assess the genetic diversity of CV Swainson's Hawks and, second, to determine whether CV Swainson's Hawks are genetically distinct from those occurring in the GBGP. Population genetic data describing contemporary genetic diversity and population structure among Swainson's Hawks provide an important compliment to previous ecological and behavioral studies.

Methods

Sample Collection

Whole blood and contour feathers were collected from 357 Swainson' s Hawks from California, east to North Dakota and Alberta, and south through Texas between 2003 and 2005, as well as five Ferruginous Hawks (*Buteo regalis*) for outgroup comparison. Samples were collected from CV, the nearest breeding populations to the north, southeast, and east as well as from five additional GBGP locations. These sampling locations allowed comparisons between CV and the remainder of the Swainson's Hawk range in GBGP as well as for comparisons of equally distant locations within GBGP. Approximately 0.2 ml blood was drawn via medial metatarsal venipuncture and two feathers were plucked from the breast. Blood samples were stored in 1.2 ml of Longmire's lysis buffer (100 mM Tris pH 8.0, 100 mM EDTA, 10 mM NaCl, 0.5% SDS) at ambient temperature until delivered to laboratory facilities where they were preserved at –80°C. Feather samples were stored in paper envelopes and kept cool and dry. Samples were collected from adults, juveniles, and pre-fledge young in nests by licensed raptor biologists and from juveniles and adults treated at several wildlife rehabilitation facilities. Wild birds were leg-banded with U.S. Geological Survey tags and either released or returned to nests. One individual per presumed family group (nestlings and parents) was included in the sampling for this study. Total cell DNA was isolated from 25 μl of blood/buffer solution or feather calamus using QIAGEN DNeasy kits (QIAGEN Inc.). DNA was stored at 4°C while in use, and then transferred to –80°C upon completion of genetic work.

Data Collection

Each individual was genotyped at 19 microsatellite loci (BswA110w, BswD122w, BswA204w, BswA317w, BswD 210w, BswD220w, BswA303w, BswB 11 law, BswD234w, BswD3 10w, BswD313w, BswB220w, BswB221w, BswD 327w, BswA302w, BswA312w, BswD107w, BswD127w, and BswD324w) using DNA extracted from whole blood in six multiplex PCRs carried out following the conditions in Hull et al. 2006. PCR products were separated with a 3730 DNA Analyzer.

A total of 416 base pairs of domain I of the mitochondrial control region were amplified via PCR using primers 16065F and H15414. Both blood and feather samples were used from the same individuals to aid in detection of nuclear-mitochondrial insertions. PCR products were prepared for sequencing reactions using Ultra-clean purification kits and submitted to the UC Davis DNA Sequencing Facility for sequencing reactions and electrophoresis using primers 14965F and H15414. Primer 14965F, TTGTACATTAACTTATATTCCACAT ATCAT, was designed specifically for this project and is located 10 base pairs downstream from a poly-c repeat that inhibited the sequencing reaction. Sequences were examined and aligned using the software SEQUENCHER.

Microsatellite Data Analysis

Samples from CV and GBGP regions were tested for deviations from Hardy-Weinberg equilibrium in the program ARLEQUIN version 3.01 using Fisher's exact test with 10,000 dememorization and 100,000 Markov chain steps. Genotypic linkage equilibrium was tested using Fisher's exact test in GENEPOP with 1,000 dememorization steps, 100 batches, and 1,000 iterations per batch. A Bonferroni correction for multiple tests was used for HWE and linkage equilibrium. The presence of null alleles was tested in MICRO-CHECKER. Scoring error was evaluated by repeating amplification and scoring for 10% of samples at all loci and calculating the frequency of disagreement between runs. Heterozygosity and number of alleles per region, CV and GBGP, were tested for in MICROSATELLITE TOOLKIT. The number of private alleles in CV and GBGP was calculated in CONVERT and allelic richness, which accounts for variation in sample sizes, was calculated in FSTAT.

The program STRUCTURE, a model-based Bayesian algorithm, was used to probabilistically cluster individuals from all sites, and separately for GBGP individuals, based upon their multilocus genotypes without using *a priori* information on sampling locality. A preliminary analysis using the admixture model with flat prior was run for 100,000 iterations with an initial burn-in of 10,000 iterations for $K = 1$ through $K = 10$. This parameter set was performed 10 times and the log $\Pr(X|K)$ statistic averaged across runs. Based upon the preliminary results, a second parameter set, using the admixture model with flat prior, burn-in of 100,000 iterations, and run length of 1,000,000 iterations, was performed and log $\Pr(X|K)$ statistic averaged across 10 runs. The most likely number of clusters, K, was chosen by determining the K value where the averaged log $\Pr(X|K)$ was maximized and subsequently selecting the minimum value for K that did not sacrifice significant explanatory power. Recently, this method has been shown to perform as well or better than the method presented by Evanno et al. 2005, especially in cases of moderate differentiation. We defined individual membership to a cluster based upon highest membership assignment probability.

Population genetic structure was further investigated by comparing the probability that each sampled individual could be genetically assigned to one of the nine sampling localities. Following a Bayesian approach, as implemented in GENECLASS2 version 2.0.b, each Swainson's Hawk sampled during the breeding season at one of the nine sampling sites was removed from the total sample of individuals and treated as an unknown and the probability of assignment to each sampling sites was determined using the Monte-Carlo resampling method of Paetkau et al. 2004.

Population differentiation between regions (CV and GBGP) and between sampling sites was estimated in ARLEQUIN using pairwise F_{ST}, following the infinite alleles model (IAM), and R_{ST}, following the step-wise mutation model (SMM) of microsatellite evolution. F_{ST} estimations can be potentially depressed by high mutation rates such as those found in many microsatellite loci. In contrast, R_{ST} is less dependent upon mutation rates. However, R_{ST} has greater variance and estimations will be compromised by deviations from the SMM, such as imperfect repeats. A Bonferroni correction for multiple tests was used to determine significance of F_{ST} and R_{ST} values among sampling locations and years.

To estimate the time required for development of observed degree of population differentiation (between region F_{ST}), a hypothetical sample with two populations (simulating CV and GBGP regions) was modeled using EASYPOP. The model parameters were as follows: monogamy, equal sex ratio, no migration, step-wise mutation model, mutation rate of 0.001, and population estimates of 1400 pairs for CV and 38000 for GBGP. All parameters were set in such a way as to generate a minimum estimate of required time since divergence. For example, the setting of no migration, while not likely to be a reflection of biological reality, helps to establish a minimum divergence time. For the same reason, the estimates of population size used are low values of the range reported in the literature. The model was run for 200 generations and 50 replicates of the model were performed. The estimated F_{ST} values were averaged across replicates and plotted against time in generations.

To investigate the potentially confounding effect of geographic distance, a Mantel test was used in ARLEQUIN to test for correlation between pairwise genetic and geographic distances. The dependent variable in this analysis was a matrix of genetic distances (expressed as $F_{ST}/(1-F_{ST})$) while the independent matrix was composed of pairwise geographic distances between centroids of sampling localities. Because the Mantel test is potentially sensitive to small sample sizes, the relationship between genetic and geographic distance was investigated in two ways: first by comparing all pairs of the nine sampling sites and then by excluding those sites that were represented by fewer than 15 samples.

Tests for evidence of recent genetic bottlenecks were performed using Wilcoxon sign-rank tests in the program BOTTLENECK using the strict IAM and a two-phase model (TPM) of microsatellite mutation which allows a user to specified proportion of the SMM into a multi-step model; we ran the TPM analysis with a setting of 70% SMM (12 of 19 loci appear to follow the SMM). A significant excess of heterozygotes is indicative of a recent population bottleneck.

Control Region Sequence Analysis

Number of variable sites, number of haplotypes, haplotype diversity, and nucleotide diversity were calculated in DNAsp. Pairwise F_{ST} values between each sampling site and between CV and GBGP regions were calculated using pairwise Juke & Cantor distances and haplotype frequencies in ARLEQUIN and significance was assessed using 10,000 permutations. A Bonferroni correction for multiple tests was used to determine significance of F_{ST} values among sampling locations and years. We tested for a correlation between genetic distance, as measured by F_{ST}, and geographic distance using a Mantel test with 100,000 permutations in ARLEQUIN. Again, comparisons were made both for all nine sample sites and those sites with 15 or greater samples (Alberta n = 13, Arizona n = 23, Central Plains n = 33, Northern Plains n = 18, Idaho n = 32, Inyo n = 12, Modoc Plateau n = 42, Utah/Nevada n=16, and CV n = 71).

Maximum likelihood and unweighted maximum parsimony trees were generated using PAUP* version 4.0b10. Bayesian analyses were performed in MRBAYES version 3.0b4. In all three analyses B. regalis was used as an outgroup. MRMODELTEST was used to identify the model of sequence evolution and parameter estimates that best fit the data. For heuristic maximum likelihood and Bayesian analyses, both hierarchical likelihood ratio and Akaike information criterion tests returned best scores for the fit of the data to the general time reversible plus invariable plus gamma model of nucleotide evolution. Maximum parsimony (100 replicate data sets) and maximum likelihood (500 replicate data sets) boot-strapping were performed in PAUP* using the same parameters as the original heuristic searches. For Bayesian analyses, the Markov Chain Monte Carlo simulation was started with a random tree. Four chains were run simultaneously for 10,000,000 generations with a tree sampled every 10,000 generations resulting in a total of 1,000 trees. Interpretation of the likelihood values indicated that the simulation achieved stability at approximately 80,000 generations. We conservatively estimated the first 250,000 generations to represent the initial burn-in; these were discarded.

Several metrics were used to investigate historical demography. The expansion coefficient (*S*/*d*), the ratio of variable sequence positions (*S*) relative to the mean number of pairwise differences between haplotypes (*d*), was calculated following Peck and Congdon (2004). Large values for *S*/*d* suggest recent population expansion while small values indicate constant population size. Mismatch distributions and raggedness statistics (rg) were calculated in DNAsp. Unimodal mismatch distributions are indicative of population expansion while a multimodal, ragged distribution of pairwise differences is more typical of a population at mutation-drift equilibrium. We also calculated Fu's F_S statistic and used Tajima's *D*-test to detect past population expansions. Fu's F_S has greater statistical power to detect population expansion than other available tests. Tajima's *D*-test compares the number of nucleotide differences between sequences and the number of differences between segregating sites; population expansion will result in a significant negative departure from zero. Fu and Li's D^* and F^* statistics were used to test for the confounding effect of background selection; significant values are associated with selection. Comparing F_S, D^*, and F^* can permit discrimination of population expansion from background selection. A significant F_S with non-significant D^* and F^* supports an interpretation of population expansion.

Of 357 total Swainson's Hawk samples collected, 306 samples were collected during the breeding season prior to dispersal and migration and thus geographic origin could be confirmed. All 357 samples were used in determination of total number of alleles and haplotypes among Swainson's Hawks, initial STRUCTURE cluster identification, construction of phylogenetic trees, and analysis of demographic history for the total Swainson's Hawk population. For all other analyses, only individuals collected during the breeding season were included in order to insure that sampled individuals were representative of local breeding populations and not migrants.

Results

Microsatellites

All 19 microsatellite loci amplified in Swainson's Hawks with no more than two alleles per individual. The 10% quality control analysis revealed a 0.3% rate of disagreement between initial and secondary scores. In CV mean observed heterozygosity was 0.81 ± 0.01 and the mean number of alleles per locus was 12.74 ± 6.90. In GBGP mean observed heterozygosity was 0.83 ± 0.01 and the mean number of alleles per locus was 16.63 ± 9.65. The number of private alleles was generally higher for GBGP than CV, however allelic richness at each locus was similar between populations.

Table 9.1. Polymorphism data for 19 Swainson's Hawk-specific microsatellite loci tested across 306 individuals

Locus	*A*	*A/locus CV*	*A/locus GBGP*	AR_C *CV*	AR_C *GBGP*
BswA1 10w	13	10 (2)	11 (3)	9.92	10.00
BswD122w	24	16 (1)	23 (8)	15.88	19.78
BswA204w	18	12	18 (6)	11.92	15.49
BswA317w	11	9 (1)	10 (2)	8.92	9.01
BswD210w	26	22	26 (4)	21.90	23.90
BswD220w	15	9	15 (6)	9.00	13.50
BswA303w	12	7	12 (5)	6.99	9.57
BswB11law	6	6 (1)	5	5.99	4.57
BswD234w	13	9	13 (4)	9.00	10.78
BswD310w	31	24	31 (7)	23.87	25.64
BswD313w	14	10	14 (4)	10.00	12.03
BswB220w	11	8	11 (3)	7.96	10.43
BswB221w	7	5	7 (2)	5.00	6.26
BswD327w	11	8 (1)	10 (3)	8.00	8.59
BswA302w	12	10 (1)	11 (2)	9.96	9.62
BswA312w	15	11	15 (4)	11.00	14.02
BswD107w	49	31 (3)	46 (18)	30.82	35.96
BswD127w	19	16 (2)	17 (3)	15.85	13.78
BswD324w	23	19 (2)	21 (3)	18.77	18.54

Preliminary STRUCTURE analyses indicated that log $Pr(X|K)$ declined sharply beyond $K = 5$, consequently the second parameter set focused on K values of 1–5. For the second parameter set, log $Pr(X|K)$, averaged across 10 runs, peaked at $K = 2$ and declined beyond $K = 3$. Geographic structure was apparent for the two clusters, with one cluster assigning primarily to GBGP and a second occurring mostly in CV with other individuals spread across GBGP. For $K = 3$ a similar geographic pattern was evident for two of the clusters, while the third cluster appeared evenly in both regions and did not provide additional explanatory value. No geographic structure was evident when GBGP individuals were analyzed separately and a graph of log $\Pr(X|K)$ peaked at $K = 1$.

Self-assignment of breeding Swainson's Hawks from nine sampling sites resulted in poor assignment to site of origin. In general, Swainson's Hawks sampled from GBGP sampling sites had a higher probability of assigning to a GBGP site than to CV. Similarly, CV individuals generally had a higher probability of assignment to CV than to any of the eight GBGP sampling sites. However, in both GBGP and CV a majority of individuals also had a low but nontrivial probability of assigning to the alternate region indicating that an origin from an alternate region could not be rejected.

Table 9.2. Average probability of individual assignment for Swainson's Hawks sampled from nine sampling localities

Source	*Average probability of assignment*								
	AB	*AZ*	*CP*	*NP*	*ID*	*IN*	*MP*	*UN*	*CV*
AB	0.17	0.13	0.19	0.08	0.08	0.05	0.10	0.42*	0.09
AZ	0.33	0.28	0.13	0.03	0.12	0.06	0.09	0.36*	0.09
CP	0.48	0.18	0.53	0.08	0.37	0.10	0.33	0.64*	0.27
NP	0.56	0.21	0.38	0.29	0.27	0.05	0.31	0.60*	0.22
ID	0.48	0.16	0.32	0.08	0.52*	0.11	0.30	0.52*	0.30
IN	0.39	0.08	0.18	0.06	0.20	0.25	0.25	0.46*	0.13
MP	0.42	0.20	0.26	0.09	0.28	0.13	0.50*	0.50*	0.30
UN	0.32	0.07	0.16	0.03	0.19	0.06	0.11	0.38*	0.08
CV	0.43	0.28	0.44	0.13	0.47	0.12	0.48	0.75	0.87*

A pairwise comparison between CV and GBGP resulted in a significant, but small F_{ST} ($F_{ST} = 0.011$, $P < 0.001$) but non-significant R_{ST} ($R_{ST} = 0.001$, $P = 0.24$). When seven of the 19 loci (BswD122w, BswD210w, BswD310w, BswD313w, BswD107w, BswD127w, BswD324w, all pentanucleotide repeats) apparently deviating from the SMM, were removed from the analysis, both F_{ST} and R_{ST} were significant between CV and GBGP ($F_{ST} = 0.014$, $P < 0.001$; $R_{ST} = 0.012$, $P = 0.002$). Pairwise F_{ST} values were significant among a majority of sampling sites while R_{ST} values were entirely nonsignificant when all 19 loci were included. Upon removal of the seven loci not conforming to the SMM, eight pairwise R_{ST} values became significant.

The model results averaged across 50 EASYPOP simulations suggested that a minimum of between 68 and 75 generations were necessary to achieve the observed degree of population differentiation (F_{ST} = 0.011) between CV and GBGP. Using a generation time of three years for Swainson's Hawks, the time in generations required to attain the observed differentiation corresponds to roughly 200 years.

No significant relationship was found between genetic and geographic distance ($P = 0.43$, $r = 0.046$) among all nine sampling sites. However, when the two sampling sites with fewer than 15 samples were removed from the analysis a significant effect of isolation-by-distance was found ($P = 0.04$, $r = 0.48$).

A significant excess of heterozygotes ($P < 0.001$ IAM, $P = 0.006$ TPM, Wilcoxon sign-rank test) was detected in the total population of Swainson's Hawks indicating a relatively recent (within the past century) range-wide bottleneck. When considered separately, a significant excess of heterozygotes was detected in both CV and GBGP suggesting that both CV($P < 0.001$ IAM, $P = 0.005$ TPM, Wilcoxon sign-rank test) and GBGP ($P < 0.001$ IAM, P = 0.002 TPM, Wilcoxon sign-rank test) regions have experienced recent bottlenecks in effective population size.

Control Region Sequences

A total of 279 control region sequences were generated following removal of individuals sampled outside the breeding season and cases of poor sequencing reactions. All sequences were archived in GenBank. No evidence of nuclear copies of the control region was observed: replicate sequences from DNA extracted from feathers and blood yielded identical sequences, and no double peaks were observed in the electropherograms. Additionally, sequences aligned with previously published *Buteo* control region sequences. Control region sequencing revealed 24 (5.7%) variable sites among Swainson's Hawks, resulting in 33 haplotypes in 416 base pairs of control region sequence among 279 Swainson' s Hawks. Of these, 21 sites were parsimony informative. Among all samples haplotype diversity was 0.608 ± 0.035 with an associated nucleotide diversity of 0.00394.

The average number of nucleotide differences among haplotypes was 1.638. Among 208 GBGP breeding samples, 28 haplotypes were identified (23 unique to GBGP) and 23 variable nucleotide positions, the average number of differences between GBGP haplotypes was 1.586.

GBGP haplotype diversity was 0.573 ± 0.041 and nucleotide diversity was 0.00381. A total of 71 CV Swainson' s Hawks yielded 8 haplotypes (3 unique to CV) among 14 variable sites with an average of 1.366 nucleotide differences between each haplotype. Haplotype and nucleotide diversity in CV were 0.590 ± 0.062 and 0.00328, respectively. Two singleton haplotypes were identified in individuals sampled outside of the breeding season.

Bootstrap analysis of maximum-likelihood and maximum parsimony trees and Bayesian posterior probabilities found 100% support for the distinction between the Swainson's Hawk clade and Ferruginous Hawks. Very limited support for differentiation among any of the Swainson's Hawk haplotypes was detected, and no geographic structure was evident. The nodes with weak bootstrap and Bayesian support do not correspond to particular regions and samples from the CV and GBGP are interspersed throughout the tree.

A minimum spanning network of all haplotypes revealed moderate structuring of haplotypes and suggested that haplotype A may have been the progenitor of the majority of Swainson's Hawk haplotypes. In contrast to GBGP, CV minimum spanning network displayed several missing intermediate haplotypes even though CV was the most extensively sampled site in the study. By combining samples from Modoc Plateau and Idaho a sample size (n = 74) similar to CV (n = 71) was achieved. The minimum spanning network of this partial GBGP data set revealed twice as many haplotypes and fewer missing steps than the CV group, suggesting the CV may have experienced a loss of haplotypes.

A pairwise comparison between CV and GBGP resulted in a non-significant F_{ST} using both haplotype frequencies and pairwise distances following Bonferroni correction (F_{ST} = 0.016, P = 0.026 and F_{ST} = 0.025, P = 0.003). Pairwise F_{ST} values were non-significant except in comparisons of Alberta with Arizona, Arizona with Northern Plains, Central Plains with Central Valley, and Alberta with Central Valley when using a pairwise distance estimate of F_{ST}. All pairwise comparisons were non-significant when using haplotype frequencies. A Mantel test failed to reveal a significant correlation between genetic and geographic distance for control region sequences when comparing all sites (P = 0.056, r = 0.333) as well as in comparison of the seven sites with greater than 15 samples (P = 0.123, r = 0.297).

We evaluated the historical demography of pooled Swainson's Hawks from all sites as well as GBGP and CV individually. In all three cases mismatch distributions closely fit the unimodal distribution expected for a recent population expansion (Total τ = 1.01, range 0.00–11.61; GBGP τ = 0.00, range 0.00–8.382; CV τ = 0.256, range 0.00–6.166) and in each case the raggedness index was low (Total rg = 0.047, $P < 0.86$; GBGP rg = 0.063, $P < 0.79$; CV rg = 0.049, P < 0.81). Tajima's D was not significant in any of the groupings examined (Total D = –1.57, $P > 0.05$; GBGP $D = -1.61$, $P = > 0.05$; CV $D = -1.52$, P> 0.10). Fu's F_S statistic was significant in the total population ($F_S = -28.437$, $P < 0.001$) and in the GBGP ($F_S = -21.824$, $P < 0.001$). In the CV, F_S was qualitatively much smaller and non-significant ($F_S = -2.120$, $P = 0.06$). Fu and Li's F^* and D^* were not significant in each case (Total $D^* = 0.379$, $P > 0.10$, $F^* = -0.521$, $P > 0.10$; GBGP $D^* = 0.427$, $P > 0.10$, $F^* = -0.475$, $P >$ 0.10; CV $D^* = 0.495$, $P > 0.10$, $F^* = -0.250$, P> 0.10) suggesting selection was not responsible for the observed pattern. Expansion coefficients for the total sample set and GBGP were found to have large values of similar magnitudes (Total S/d = 15.96; GBGP S/d = 14.50), while the expansion coefficient was somewhat smaller in for CV (S/d = 10.25).

Discussion

Genetic Diversity and Population Structure

Genetic data from multi-locus microsatellite genotypes suggests that Swainson's Hawks are subdivided into two clusters with one cluster primarily occurring in the Great Basin, Great Plains, and southwestern deserts (GBGP) and a second cluster found mostly in the California Central Valley (CV) with several individuals spread across the GBGP. The observed heterozygosity was quite high and similar between the GBGP and CV as was allelic richness at each locus while a greater number of private alleles occurred in the GBGP than in the CV.

The overall genetic differentiation between GBGP and CV appears limited in absolute terms (as indicated by pairwise F_{ST} estimates) and is additionally accompanied by a pattern of isolation by distance. The self-assignment of individuals generally assigned samples to their region of origin (GBGP or CV) but not to individual sampling site. Many samples also had a low, but not negligible, probability of assigning to the alternate region, reflecting an overall low degree of differentiation between regions. Simulated populations help to provide a context for interpreting the low level of observed differentiation.

The simulation conservatively suggests that this degree of differentiation would require approximately 200 years to develop; a timeframe corresponding roughly with European settlement of western North America. Given the number of parameters that were estimated for the model, the precision of this estimate may be limited. However, the parameters were estimated purposefully in a way to minimize time since divergence (e.g., no migration). The resulting simulation data do indicate that the observed differentiation would not be achieved in a few generations, suggesting that the degree of differentiation observed may not be due to short-term stochastic fluctuations in Swainson's Hawk populations.

Interpretation of the significant, yet low, differentiation observed in the microsatellite data should be undertaken with caution. Considering the large sample sizes used here and the number of highly polymorphic markers employed, this study had high statistical power to detect fine-scale population differentiation. Thus, very small differences between populations may be detected as statistically significant although differences may not be biologically meaningful. Among Swainson's Hawks, differentiation between CV and GBGP is lower than reported in a previous investigation of clearly isolated island populations of Galapagos Hawks, phylogenetically the closest relative of Swainson' s Hawks, using minisatellite data (F_{ST} = 0.017–0.896). While different types of molecular markers were employed, and the population size of the two species is drastically different, the difference in observed differentiation between Swainson's Hawks and Galapagos Hawks suggests that Swainson's Hawks have yet to reach the same level of isolation as found between island populations of Galapagos Hawks.

The absence of significant mitochondrial differentiation between CV and GBGP along with quite low values for F_{ST} between sampling sites indicates no population structure is present among mitochondrial control region lineages. Similar pairwise measures of F_{ST} were found between sampling sites in a continent-wide study of White-bellied Sea-Eagles in Australia (F_{ST} = 0–0.126) where a high level of population connectivity was documented. The absence of a correlation between genetic and geographic distance indicates that Swainson's Hawks are effectively panmictic with respect to the mitochondrial genome. As an effectively single non-recombining marker, the control region sequence data may not have enough statistical power to detect population structure at low levels.

Historical Demography

For the total population and GBGP, control region sequences reveal a recent population expansion in Swainson's Hawks. Evidence of expansion is inferred from the close fit of mismatch distributions with theoretical expectations, low nucleotide diversities accompanied by high haplotype diversities, large expansion coefficients, significant FS statistic, and star-like minimum spanning networks and control region phylogeny. The CV data are more complex with expansion suggested by the mismatch distribution and large expansion coefficient, but not by the F_s statistic which was non-significant and much smaller than in the total population and GBGP. The non-significant values obtained for Fu and Li's F^* and D^* statistics in all comparisons suggest that the observed patterns are not a consequence of background selection.

Considering the range of reported mutation rates for the avian control region domain I, the limited raptor fossil record available for estimating a Swainson's Hawk specific mutation rate, and error associated with expansion statistics, determining timing of a possible population expansion with accuracy would be difficult.

Previous studies of North American taxa have frequently detected signals of population expansion associated with the most recent glacial maxima approximately 18,000 years ago. Retreat of glacial ice clearly provided Swainson's Hawks with the opportunity to occupy the northern plains and may have resulted in the signature of population expansion seen in control region data for the total population and GBGP.

The microsatellite data provides an interesting contrast to the evidence of population expansion seen in the mitochondria. For both CV and GBGP a significant excess of heterozygotes indicates that Swainson's Hawks have experienced recent population bottlenecks. The bottlenecks are likely associated with declines occurring during the 19th and 20th centuries as human settlement resulted in increased habitat loss and direct mortality.

A severe population reduction among California Swainson's Hawks may have been responsible for the loss of control region haplotypes as indicated by the contrasting CV and partial GBGP minimum spanning networks, eight haplotypes versus 16 haplotypes. A loss of haplotypes may have consequently reduced the signal of previous population expansion.

Conservation Implications

The highly polymorphic microsatellite loci employed here resulted in an observed heterozygosity of 0.81 for CV Swainson's Hawks. Using less polymorphic loci, previous studies have observed lower heterozygosity in several raptor species ranging from 0.099 in the Mauritius Kestrel (*Falco punctatus*) to 0.6 14 in the Lesser Kestrel

(*F. naumanni*). The high level of observed heterozygosity at microsatellite loci among Swainson's Hawks occurring in CV belies the apparent loss of rare alleles which suggests that some evolutionary potential may have been lost. This assertion cannot be established definitively without a comparative sample collected prior to the bottleneck. In parallel with loss of rare microsatellite alleles, the minimum spanning network for CV suggests that several intermediate haplotypes may have been lost as a consequence of population decline.

The absence of both reciprocally monophyletic groups in control region data and significant allele frequency differences indicates that the Swainson's Hawks in CV do not meet the standards proposed by Moritz (1994) for an evolutionarily significant unit. The pattern suggested by the data is one of effective panmixia for control region and limited differentiation for the microsatellite loci. As discussed above, interpretation of weak differentiation between Swainson' s Hawk populations can be challenging.

The observed divergence may reflect either an absence of population structure or incipient divergence, as seen in the analysis of simulated populations. Incipient divergence may be associated with recent changes observed in migratory behavior, a highly plastic trait, among CV Swainson's Hawks. In contrast to the GBGP, where over-wintering Swainson's Hawks have not been documented, Swainson's Hawks in CV have recently established a winter population. This change in behavior, along with the use of coastal western Mexico as wintering range by CV Swainson's Hawks, may reflect an ecological response to changing environmental conditions, possibly local agriculture practices or climatic changes. Such changes in behavior could ultimately contribute to nascent divergence in Swainson's Hawks.

As demonstrated by their migratory abilities, Swainson's Hawks are clearly capable of long distance dispersal which might preclude the formation of population structure. The limited dispersal observed among adults and juveniles in California suggests that these birds may not mix as readily with individuals from other regions potentially allowing genetically distinct populations to emerge. The mechanism limiting dispersal within California Swainson' s Hawks is not understood.

While the genetic data is somewhat ambiguous relative to distinct population segments, differences between CV and GBGP in traits with potential fitness consequences, such as migratory behavior and morphology, along with a precipitous decline in numbers in California call for careful conservation, management, and monitoring of Swainson's

Hawks of the Central Valley. If populations are allowed to continue to decline and fragment, genetic diversity may be lost at an ever increasing rate as has been observed previously in raptors, and ultimately require an expensive and time consuming recovery effort. Continued efforts should be directed towards monitoring of census population size in the Central Valley, determination of population trends, periodic evaluation of genetic diversity and population structure as census numbers change, and habitat conservation.

10

GENETICS OF CANINE BEHAVIOR

Behavior is a result of nature (genetics) and nurture (learning or experience). We shall review the history of canine behavioral genetics and explore the latest findings. The publication of the canine genome allows us to make some inferences.

FOXES

One of the most thorough studies of canid behavioral genetics deals with foxes, not dogs. Selection for a tame and for an aggressive strain of silver foxes over 30 years by Dmitry Belyaev and Lyudmila Trut resulted in large differences in behavior and in morphology. The tame foxes were more likely to have spots, floppy ears, and curly tails. Tame and aggressive foxes have been bred and there are 300 backcross offspring. These three generation pedigrees are allowing Anna Kukekova and her colleagues at Cornell University to use linkage analysis to find the gene for tameness and for aggression. The karyotypic differences between fox and dog represent 26 chromosomal fusion and four fission events, so that anything learned about foxes will apply to dogs as well.

Breed Differences in Behavior

There are several approaches to classifying behaviors. We shall review four of these: breed differences in behavioral neoteny; breed differences in social signaling; breed differences in prevalence of behavior problems; and opinions of dog experts on behavioral characteristics of various breeds.

There are obvious physical differences among dog breeds and, although behavior does not vary as widely as size and skeletal features, there are marked breed differences in behavior. In fact, many lectures on canine genetics begin with a statement about genetic differences in behavior, but few of the genes are known. Dr. Yukari Takeuchi and her colleagues at Tokyo University have made the most progress and we will review their findings here.

What are the different genotypes of dogs? Genetically, dogs can be placed in four clusters. The most genetically distinct are the Asian breeds: Chow, Akita, and sled dogs, such as the Husky. The second cluster includes the guard dogs, mastiffs, bull dog, boxer and Bernese mountain dog. The third cluster consists of herding breeds, the collie, and Shetland sheepdog, and some of the sight hounds, including the greyhound. The remaining cluster includes modern hunting breeds including gun dogs, hounds, and terriers. It is surprising that the Western breeds sort out genetically close to the American Kennel Club classifications. For example, the mastiff, bull dogs, pitbulls, and boxers, etc. are closely related to one another. The aggression noted in these breeds can certainly be explained as genetic. Rottweilers do not belong to that group despite their brachycephalic features. The hounds are closely related, as are the terriers.

Beagle, Basenji, Cocker Spaniel, Wire Haired Fox Terrier, and Shetland Sheepdog. The earliest and still most complete study of breed differences in canine behavior was performed by Scott and Fuller (1974) at Jackson Laboratory in Maine. This group, who also discovered the critical periods of socialization in dogs, studied five breeds: cocker spaniels, wire haired fox terriers, basenjis, Shetland sheepdogs, and beagles. The five breeds were tested for their ability to learn three types of tasks: forced training, reward training, and problem solving.

The forced method of training was used to teach the dogs to sit still on a scale, to heel on a leash, and to stay and jump on command. In all three types of tasks, the cocker spaniels ranked highest in correct performance. The trainability of cockers in these situations is probably the result of selection within the breed for dogs that would crouch in response to a hand signal. Although cockers are not often used for hunting now, the behavioral predisposition remains.

All the dogs learned to heel within the 10-day training period, but there were marked differences in the types of errors that dogs of the various breeds made in the early sessions. Basenjis fought the leash and often pulled ahead or lagged behind; Shetland sheepdogs interfered with the trainer, that is, tangled the leash around his legs. Beagles vocalized in protest. The breed differences in performance were evident on the first training trials and persisted, even though all the dogs improved.

Reward training consisted of showing the dog a piece of fish in a box and then restraining the puppy behind a wire gate before allowing him to run to the box and eat the fish. The position of the box was changed to measure goal orientation versus habit formation. Basenjis performed best on this test, probably because they could run the fastest. With the additional trials, all the dogs reduced the time they took to reach the reward. When motor skills of the five breeds were compared, the basenji was also best.

Problem solving was also studied. The first type of problem the dogs were supposed to solve was a barrier or detour. The dogs were separated from a food reward by a wire barrier. When they learned to run around a short barrier, the barrier was extended and later formed into a U-shape to increase the difficulty of the problem. The dogs were only 6 weeks of age and had considerable difficulty in solving the barrier problem that an adult dog could master easily. The puppies often yelped, and it was noted that they never solved the problem while yelping, but instead engaged in stereotypic activity. Few puppies did well on the barrier test, but basenjis, which are already active at 6 weeks, did best. Puppies of other breeds still tend to be fat and clumsy at 6 weeks and would react to failure by going to sleep.

Another type of problem was a manipulation test in which the dogs were tested for their ability to pull a dish of food from under a box by pawing or pulling it out with their noses. Later, the dish was positioned in such a way that it could be maneuvered out from under the box only by pulling on a dowel and string attached to the dish. Again, the basenjis were the most successful. When maze learning was tested in RLLRRR (right, left, left, and so on) or LRLL mazes, beagles did best. They completed the maze most quickly and made the fewest errors.

A final test of problem-solving behavior, when the dogs were 22 weeks old, was a delayed response test in which the dogs were shown a visual cue that indicated which side of a T- maze led to freedom. Before the dog was allowed to run the maze, a delay from 1 to 240 seconds was imposed. As in all problem solving, there were great individual differences, but cocker spaniels could remember after the longest delay, and Shetland sheepdogs had the poorest memory.

The extensive studies at Jackson Laboratory indicate that care must be taken in comparing intelligence, even within a species, since breeds of dogs differ markedly in their relative performance depending on the task to be learned.

The most intriguing result was the interaction of genotype and experience. Puppies were raised in isolation and exposed to either tolerant humans or disciplinary humans who made the puppies sit and wouldn't play with them. Later the puppies were presented one by one with a bowl of food. If they approached, the handler would clap his hands to frighten them away. The handler then left the room so the puppies were free to eat the food. The basenjiis did, no matter how they had been handled. The Shetland sheepdog never did, no matter how they had been handled. The disciplined beagles ate the food, but not the tolerantly treated ones. The conclusion is that identical handling will have different effects on different genotypes of dogs.

Border Collies and Newfoundlands

At the University of California at Berkeley, Jasper Rine and Elaine Ostrander crossed border collies and Newfoundlands. The F_1 generation were bred to one another and in the F_3 generation, the various behavior traits associated with each breed-retrieving and giving eye (staring at sheep or person) for border collies, and love of water and friendliness of Newfoundlands were inherited separately, so that some dogs loved water like Newfoundlands and gave eye like border collies.

Nervous Pointers

At the University of Arkansas, selective breeding for five generations resulted in two strains of pointers - a nervous (E) and a normal strain (A). The former are much more difficult to train and the tricyclic anti-depressant imipramine does not improve their behavior. The results indicate that nervousness or aversion is a result of additive gene action. The A dogs are friendly, active, people-seeking dogs, whereas the E are nervous, exhibit marked timidity, reduced activity, little exploratory behavior and nearly catatonic immobility when people are nearby. Their heart rate is markedly reduced and their eyes are directionally fixed.

Deafness can be diagnosed behaviorally by observing a dog's response to a sudden noise. This is easiest to do when the dog is panting in a warm environment. He will interrupt his panting if he hears the sound. A more quantitative method is the brainstem auditory evoked response (BAER). A speaker is placed in the dog's ear and sound played through it. Recordings are made from electrodes placed on the neck over the hindbrain.

In a normally hearing dog, a change in voltage will occur in every synapse from the auditory nucleus to the cortex - eight in all. If the dog is deaf, there will be no change in voltage. Sounds may be played at various decibels, to detect partial deafness and at various frequencies. Using BAER technology, Steinberg et al. (1994) have detected an autosomal recessive deafness in some of the nervous pointers. The relationship of the auditory problem to the nervous behavior is unknown, but appears insufficient to explain the behavior.

Expert Opinion of Breed Behavior Differences

The largest study of opinions of breed differences is that of Hart and Miller (1985). They surveyed 48 veterinarians and 48 obedience judges as to 13 traits in 56 breeds of dog. The thirteen characteristics were: excitability; general activity; snapping at children; excessive barking; demand for affection; territorial defense; watchdog barking; aggression toward other dogs; dominance over the owner; aptitude for obedience training; ease of house breaking; destructiveness; and playfulness. The breeds were ranked by decile. Dogs in the tenth decile rank higher than 90% of other breeds for that characteristic. Those in the first decile rank below all the other breeds in that characteristic. Let us compare three breeds: the beagle, golden retriever and German shepherd.

The beagle ranks in the eighth decile for excitability, the ninth for general activity, the fifth for snapping at children, the ninth for excessive barking, and the third for demand for affection, the third for territorial defense, the fourth for watchdog barking, the fifth for aggression toward other dogs, the eighth for dominance over the owner, the first for obedience training and ease of house breaking, the seventh for destructiveness, and the fifth for playfulness. The beagle is hard to obedience train and housebreak, barks a lot, and is inclined to be dominant over the owner.

The German shepherd ranks in the fifth decile for excitability, the fourth for general activity, the fifth for snapping at children, the sixth for excessive barking, the third for demand for affection, the ninth for territorial defense and watchdog barking, the eighth for aggression toward other dogs, the seventh for dominance over the owner, the ninth for obedience training, and the eighth for ease of house breaking, the ninth for destructiveness, and the seventh for playfulness. German shepherds are good watch dogs and easy to train, but destructive and inclined to be dominant over the owner.

The golden retriever ranks in the second decile for excitability, the fourth for general activity, the first for snapping at children and for excessive barking, and the seventh for demand for affection, the first for territorial defense, the third for watchdog barking, the first for aggression toward other dogs and dominance over the owner, the ninth for obedience training, and the sixth for ease of house breaking, the first for destructiveness, and the eighth for playfulness. Golden retrievers are trainable and playful, but not aggressive.

Principle components analysis revealed 3 factors - reactivity, aggressiveness, trainability – and a fourth factor that included playfulness and destructiveness. Cluster analysis of breeds with similar traits revealed seven clusters. It is interesting that snapping at children clusters with reactivity, not with aggression. They also found that those surveyed believed that there were large differences between intact males and females in behavioral traits. Females were more trainable and males were more aggressive.

Bradshaw et al. (1996) performed a similar study in which veterinarians and dog-care professionals rated various breeds of dogs on a 13 point scale. Factor analysis revealed three traits: aggressivity, reactivity, and immaturity. This resulted in eight groups which did not correspond to the breed groupings.

Dog breeds are typically divided according to historical usage into Working, Hunting, Herding, Hound and Terrier groups plus the toy group, and, in some countries, a separate Gun dog group. When the results of a temperament test involving reactions to strangers who attempt to play tug of war with the dog are compared to the historical use of the dog (for guarding, hunting, etc.), there is little correlation, but there is a similarity in response within a breed. Most interesting is that two of the most popular breeds, the Labrador and the golden retriever, the latter is fearful, the Labrador bold. These results suggest that the present use of a dog differs from the historical use.

Breed Differences in Neoteny

Coppinger and Schneider (1995) compared breeds on both behavioral and physical characteristics which they believe co-evolved. Some have puppy-like facial features - short nose and full cheeks, whereas German shepherds are fully adult with long noses and narrow cheeks. They ranked the breeds by developmental stages: heelers (huskies and corgis), headers-stalkers (collies), object players (hounds, retrievers, and poodles), and adolescents. These sheep guarding dogs show juvenile behavior, such as play, and lack mature sexual behavior.

Breed Differences in Communication

Goodwin et al. (1997) examined breed differences in signaling. They observed wolves and listed the signals they observed such as growl, stand over and stare, crouch, and submissive grin. Ten breeds of dogs were compared to wolves. These dogs lived in same breed groups, ranging in size from four to seven. They were observed for several hours and the behaviors they exhibited compared to those of wolves. Siberian huskies were most like wolves; Labrador retrievers were the next most wolf-like. At the bottom were cavalier King Charles spaniels, Norfolk terriers, and French bull dogs. The authors interpreted this as meaning that behaviors had been lost with domestication due to paedomorphosis.

Breed Differences in Behavior Problems

The statistics on deaths caused by dogs allows one to determine breed differences in aggression. Between 1979 and 1998, pitbulls killed the greatest number of people followed by Rottweilers, German shepherds, huskies, malamutes, Dobermans, and chows. These are all large breed dogs, but other popular large breeds such as Labradors and golden retrievers are not on the list. It is most interesting that Rottweilers have overtaken pitbulls and now kill more people per year. The number of Rottweilers registered had increased 5-fold between 1979 and 1998, but the number of fatalities increased seven times. The statement is often made that popularity ruins the breed, but what probably happens is that while the percentage of aggressive dogs within a breed remains the same, the total numbers increase so there are more aggressive dogs of that particular breed.

Unfortunately, these statistics and the tendency of people to sue if bitten have led homeowner insurance companies to refuse policies to people who own pitbulls or Staffordshire terriers, Rottweilers, chows, and dobermans. Breed-specific legislation has been enacted in only a few communities, but the insurance companies are essentially doing that throughout the USA.

We have been interested in aggression by dogs toward their owners. Although many breeds (Doberman pinschers, Rottweilers, German shepherds) have been selected for aggression to humans, toward vermin (terriers) or toward game, (the Japanese bear dogs, otter hounds) etc., none have been selected to bite the hand that feeds them. There is a breed that has developed this trait - the English springer spaniel (ESS). This is a serious problem and led us to try to search for the gene for aggression. There was a similar aggressive problem in Bernese

Mountain dogs, but the breeders were able to select against it and essentially eliminate the problem.

There are breed differences in the behaviors for which dogs are referred to clinical animal behaviorists. Borchelt (1983) classified the types of aggression he treated in his urban consultations. Dominance aggression was most common in English springer spaniels, doberman pinschers, toy poodles, and Lhasa apsos. Possessive aggression was most common in cocker spaniels. Protective aggression was most common in German shepherds, but fear aggression was also common in that breed, as well as in cocker spaniels and miniature poodles.

Of course, breed differences in prevalence have to be compared with the numbers of dogs of each breed in the catchment area. When comparing a private practice in Ontario, a private practice in Kansas, and a university clinic in upstate New York, Landsberg (1991) found that English springer spaniels were most often presented to the eastern clinics but not to the midwestern one. Two other behavior problems - separation anxiety and thunder phobia - revealed no breed differences. Historically, ESS present with dominance-related aggression more than would be predicted by regional breed distributions and by national breed registration statistics.

The reaction of the dog to threats to its personal space or to attempts to take a coveted object from him are more likely to reveal owner-directed aggression. A behavior screen originally developed by Victoria Voith is an invaluable tool in understanding the dog's personality. For example, the dog's response to food in his proximity, both his usual ration and human food, may be no response, a growl, a snap, or a bite. The owner checks the appropriate box - and most owners are honest because they want the dog to be better. The dog's reaction to being approached when on the bed or couch, to having its leash or collar touched, or to any reprimand is also telling. A classical form of aggression is toward one member of the family, usually the male, when he approaches the dog and wife who are on the bed or couch. This may be mate guarding or a form of possessive aggression in which the woman is the possession. Questions are also asked about the dog's reaction while on and off leash to strange humans and dogs.

The responses of aggressive ESS on the aggression screen used at Cornell University Animal Behavior Clinic were distinct from the responses of aggressive dogs of other breeds. When frequency scores for ESS and non-ESS aggressive dogs were compared across the aggression screen, the responses for ESS and non-ESS diverged on a subset of questions related to dominance, feeding, and territoriality. When analyzed by subscales, aggressive ESS were not different from other aggressive dogs except on three subscales. Aggressive ESS were not different from control ESS in severity on the child-directed and territorial aggression subscales, although aggressive non-ESS scored significantly higher than controls on both. Conversely, aggressive ESS were more severe on the food related aggression subscale, while aggressive non-ESS were not different from controls.

The comparison of aggressive ESS and other breeds of aggressive dogs found a clear distinction in responses to dominance and food-related situations (ESS more frequent than non-ESS) and to territorial situations (non-ESS more frequent than ESS).

Reisner et al. (2005) reported in a survey of over 2000 ESS that 65% of ESS with a history of biting (27% of total ESS) had bitten a familiar person, indicating that dominance-related aggression is more frequent than territoriality-related aggression among ESS. The fact that dominance-related aggression and territorial aggression can be dissociated between ESS and non-ESS, as the Golden and Reisner studies reveal, suggests that they are two distinct types of aggression.

There is a syndrome in English cocker spaniels very similar to that seen in English springer spaniels. The dogs are most likely to bite their owners. Most affected dogs are male. In this case, there is a coat color association - red cockers are most likely to bite followed by black, and then parti-colored.

Heritability

There have been several studies of heritability of traits in dogs. Heritability is the proportion of variation of a trait that can be explained by genetics.

Hunting Dogs

The traits important for hunting have been examined - pointing, nose use, search and retrieval.

Heritability of a hunting behavior was investigated by the Swedish Flatcoated Retriever club, as well as to investigate the existence of broader personality traits. During the test, the dog was exposed to various standardized hunting situations and the intensity of its reactions was scored in a test protocol by approved test leaders. The data consisted of observations for 10 traits on approximately 800-1150 dogs (depending on trait) and for two additional traits recently added to the test (with only about 190 observations). The dogs were tested in the period from 1992 to 2000. Almost all traits were affected by the test leader, the test object (dummy or game) and previous experience, whereas age and sex affected fewer of the reactions. Heritability estimates for the 10 traits were generally between 0.1 and 0.4, with an outlier of 0.74, and several of the traits were highly genetically correlated. A factor analysis on estimated breeding values revealed three factors which were interpreted as broader personality traits named: excitement, willingness to retrieve, and independence. These personality traits had heritabilities of 0.49, 0.28, and 0.16, respectively, and were weakly genetically correlated with each other (from -0.08 to 0.15).

Heritability of hunting performance of gun dogs in Norway was tested. Dogs were tested individually and performances of seven traits were judged by scores from 1 to 6. The traits are: hunting eagerness, speed, style, independence, seeking width, ability to work in the field, and cooperation. In addition, the number of birds found in the test was recorded. Genetic parameters for three breeds, German short-haired pointer, German wire-haired pointer, and Brittany spaniel were estimated. The estimated heritabilities for the scored hunting performance traits varied from $h^2 = 0.06$ to 0.28. The genetic correlations between some of the performance traits were estimated to be higher than the phenotypic correlations and were close to 1.0.

Results of field trials revealed that Finnish Hounds were found to have the highest heritability scores for pursuit and tongueing (vocalization while in pursuit of a hare or fox).

Working Dogs

Ruefenacht et al. (2002) calculated the heritability of temperament of Swiss army dogs to be low based on seven traits. The traits were: (1) affability (tested by having an unknown person approach the dog); (2) disposition for self defense (an unknown person attacks the dog); (3) disposition for self defense and defense of the handler (tested by having an unknown person attack the dog and the handler); (4) disposition for fighting in a playful manner (tested by asking the dog to fight for a sleeve or a stick); (5) courage (tested by having a man-shaped figure approach the dog); (6) ability to meet with sudden, strong auditory stimuli (tested by firing a gun at a distance and by making noise with tin cans just behind the dog); (7) disposition for forgetting unpleasant episodes (tested by scaring the dog at a certain location and then asking the dog to pass the location again); and adaptiveness to different environments and situations (tested by observations throughout the test). The estimate of heritability of these traits was low.

Of most interest to us is heritability of aggression. MacKenzie et al. (1985) examined the scores of German shepherd dogs used for attack work during World War II. The heritability of temperament was determined using 575 German shepherd dogs from the Division of Biosensor Research of the US Army. The specifics of the temperament test were not mentioned, but were all determined by one person and composite scores were used to predict future performance and indicated the animal's ability to chase and attack a decoy, and to use its sense of smell. The hip dysplasia scores also were assigned by one person. There was a negative correlation between temperament and hip dysplasia scores.

MacKenzie et al (1985) found from the scores of the dogs on their temperament tests and their pedigrees that aggressiveness - that is suitability - in an attack or sentry dog was heritable at 0.51. He also found that the best scores were associated with the worse hip scores. More recent work did not find this pattern, so the genes for the two conditions must not be closely linked.

Heritability of various behaviors of German shepherd puppies bred to be working dogs in Sweden by Wilsson and Sundgren (1998) was tested. The test was divided into two parts: fetch and retrieve, and vocalization. Willingness to retrieve objects in general was considered a good measurement of cooperativeness. Willingness to play tug of war and to approach a stranger were also evaluated.

The scores of 630 German shepherd puppies tested at eight weeks of age were used to calculate heritability. The heritability of the puppy's response was highest for activity (0.53), tug of war (0.48), and contact (0.42). Other estimates of heritability range from 0.20 to 0.27. Higher estimates on dam than on sire were found for shriek, contact, tug of war, activity, and objects visited. This indicates the environmental effect.

Pet Dogs Aggression to Owner

Of course, what is good temperament for an attack dog is not necessarily good temperament for a pet dog. In fact, most of the commonly used temperament tests rely on the dog's reaction to strange people and dogs and do not measure the reaction of the dogs to challenges by the owner. Another problem is that dogs may take a test, such as the Canine Good Citizenship test, when the dog is a year old, but the dog can become aggressive as most at genetic risk do, at two years of age.

Dominance

The Campbell Test was conducted to assess dominant behavior in puppies. The test consisted of five parts and must be conducted at the age of six to eight weeks old. Puppies were subjected to the test individually with no other person, animal or object present that could distract them. The tester, who had not seen the puppy previously, remained impassive and showed no signs of emotion throughout the test. The five parts of the test included: social attraction, following, restraint, social dominance (petting), and elevation dominance (picking up).

The Campbell test applied to 51 seven week old English cocker spaniel puppies, the offspring of four sires and 10 dams, revealed a hierarchy of dominance of 0.20 based on sire and heritability estimated on the dam of 0.46, indicating both genetic and environmental influences. It is particularly interesting that seven week old puppies demonstrate the same differences due to coat color and sex as adult English cocker spaniels, that is solid color and male puppies are more dominant than particolor and female puppies.

There is high heritability of aggression – at least in adult Golden retrievers, with heritability estimates of scores of 0.9 for aggression toward strangers.

Liinamo et al. (2007) used Restricted Maximum Likelihood method to determine heritability of aggression using the dog owner's impression of the animal's human and dog-directed aggression or the responses on the Canine Behavioral Assessment and Research Questionnaire (CBARQ). They found heritability of 0.77 for human-directed aggression and 0.81 for dog-directed aggression. There is little correlation between the two types of aggression indicating separate genetic causes of the traits. There were high heritability estimates on several CBARQ items such as strange dog approaching leashed dog (0.85), family member grooming dog (0.83), family member approaching eating dog (0.94), family member removing food (0.95), stranger trying to touch dog (0.99).

These studies indicate that dominance behavior and aggression are under genetic control and have encouraged research in the genetics of canine aggression and other misbehaviors.

Genes and Behavior

The hunt for the gene involved in aggression is very difficult. For example, one may select one neurotransmitter - for example serotonin, and determine genetic difference between aggressive and non-aggressive dogs. The difference between aggressive and non-aggressive dogs could be due to a gene controlling synthesis of the neurotransmitter, reuptake of the neurotransmitter, the enzymes that inactivate the neurotransmitter, or genes that control expression of any of the above genes.

Neurotransmitters–Dopamine

Dopamine is a neurotransmitter frequently affected by veterinary drugs. For example, acepromazine is a blocker of dopamine receptors and is used for sedation. There is an association between novelty seeking in humans and the long form of the D4 dopamine receptor. Dopamine is inactivated by an enzyme, monoamine oxidase. Aggression can occur in humans with a particular mutation of the enzyme.

Serotonin (5-Hydroxytryptamine 5-HT)

Genes involved in serotonin's production and that of its receptors are promising candidates in the genetic control of aggression. Lesch et al. (1996) found an association between anxiety and polymorphism in the serotonin transporter gene. Saudou et al. (1994) found that mice lacking the 5-HT 1β receptor for serotonin were more aggressive to strange mice, which is a behavior analogous to territorial aggression in dogs. Conversely, mice lacking the receptor for substance P, the neurotransmitter that modulates sensitivity to pain, were less aggressive to strange mice.

There is considerable evidence in primates, rodents, and dogs that aggressive individuals have lower cerebrospinal levels of 5-hydroxyindole acetic acid and homovanillic acid, the major metabolites of serotonin and dopamine respectively. Furthermore, drugs that block the reuptake of serotonin such as amitriptyline and fluoxetine decrease aggression in dogs, as well as in other species.

Norepinephrine

Alpha 2 adrenergic receptors appear to modulate aggression because knockout mice lacking the alpha2c receptors were more aggressive to strangers.

Genes and Aggression

There are many studies in mice demonstrating that certain genes influence aggression, whether any of these are involved in canine aggression remains to be determined.

Targeted disruption of a single gene - a knock out - is a powerful tool with which to study behavior in laboratory mice. Knock out of the estrogen receptor reduces aggression in female mice. Neuronal nitric oxide is involved in many reactions; knock out of the neuronal nitric oxide synthetase gene increases aggression. Knock out of the gene for alpha calcium calmodulin kinase II in tailless mice also results in aggression.

A gene coding for steroid sulfatase is located on the Y chromosome and the levels of enzyme are correlated with aggression against intruder male mice. Mice with smaller infra pyramidal mossy fiber terminal fields due to a one gene mutation were more aggressive.

Genes and Canine Behavior

There have been several promising candidate genes for canine aggression. These include the dopamine D4 receptor, the long form of which is associated with risk seeking behavior in humans and monoamoine oxidase A, an enzyme which breaks down dopamine and a mutation of which is associated with incarceration of humans, if they had a bad childhood environment.

The results of the candidate gene approach to canine aggression have been uniformly disappointing so far. Although Nimi and colleagues (1999) showed that a usually gentle breed of dog, the golden retriever, had the short form of the dopamine D4 receptor and the territorially aggressive Shiba has the long form, this is not associated with behavior but rather with the genetic differences between an Asian and an Anglo-American breed.

Van den Berg et al. (2003; 2005; 2006) investigated 4 genes involved in serotonin function: serotonin receptor 1A, (htr1A); serotonin receptor 1B (htr1B); and serotonin receptor 2A (htr2A); serotonin transporter gene (slc6A4). Linkage analysis of pedigrees of Golden retrievers did not demonstrate that any of these genes were linked with aggression.

The laboratory of Veterinary Ethology of Tokyo University has made the most progress in locating putative genes affecting canine behavior. They have obtained blood samples from five breeds of dogs: golden retriever, Labrador retriever, Maltese, miniature schnauzer, and Shiba for a total of 266 samples. They have systematically searched for differences in single nucleotide polymorphisms in genes for neurotransmitters, the enzymes that synthesize them or destroy them, and the receptors. They have compared the differences in genotype with the differences in behavior in the breeds as found by Hart and Hart (1985) and Hart and Miller (1985). The details are given below.

Hashizume et al. (2003) determined the full-length nucleotide sequences of cDNA for canine monoamine oxidase type A (MAOA) and type B (MAOB) genes that were isolated from the canine brain cDNA library. Oligonucleotide primers for PCR were constructed based on the conserved sequences reported thus far for other mammalian species. The nucleotide sequences had open reading frames of 1584 and 1563 bp for MAOA and MAOB, respectively. Both of these genes showed relatively high homology with other species in both nucleotide (> 81%) and deduced amino acid (> 85%) sequences. In Northern blot analyses, MAOA mRNA was expressed broadly in various parts of the canine brain, whereas MAOB mRNA was found only in specific brain regions, such as the hypothalamus, hippocampus, brain stem and olfactory bulb.

These results suggested that MAOA and MAOB mRNAs have subtype-specific expression patterns in the canine brain. Because mutations in monoamine oxidase have been associated with aggression in humans, these canine mutations should be examined in aggressive and non-aggressive dogs. Hashizume et al. (2005) found that 90% of Golden retrievers – a friendly breed – had the T allele of the MAOB gene, whereas the more aggressive and excitable Schnauzers had less than 90%.

Masuda et al. (2004a) identified the canine catecholamine o-methyl transferase (COMT) gene fragment and found its genetic distribution among five representative canine breeds: retriever, Labrador retriever, Maltese, miniature schnauzer, and Shiba. The amplified gene consisted of 663 bp nucleotides and was 84% homologous with the human COMT gene. Single nucleotide polymorphisms, guanine adenine substitution, were observed at the 39th (G39A), 216th (G216A) and 482nd (G482A) nucleotides. From the genotyping of the 216th polymorphism among 266 dogs by the polymerase chain reaction-restriction fragment length polymorphism method with restriction enzyme EagI, and that of the 482nd polymorphism with restriction enzyme SfcI, interbreed variations of genotypes as well as of allelic frequencies were found for both of these polymorphic regions. The G/G genotypes was dominant in the five breeds tested – golden retriever, Maltese, miniature schnauzer, and Shiba, but Labrador retriever and miniature schnauzer had more A alleles. Territorial defense is higher in Labrador retrievers and miniature schnauzers than in Maltese and golden retrievers.

Masuda et al. (2004b) searched for polymorphisms of serotonin receptors in the dog and compared allelic frequencies for the canine 5-HTR1B, 5-HTR2A, and 5-HTR2C genes among five canine breeds. The canine genes consisted of the following: 5-HTR1B, 1170 bp; 5-

HTR2A, 1413 bp; and 5-HTR2C, 1377 bp. All of these genes were highly homologous with the human genes. There were no polymorphisms in the 5-HTR2A, and 5-HTR2C genes. They found six single nucleotide polymorphisms (SNPs) in the 5- HTR1B gene (G57A, A157C, G246A, C660G, T955C, and G1146C). Genotyping of the respective SNPs revealed that there were inter-breed variations in the genotypes and allelic frequencies for four out of the six identified SNPs. The G57A and A1 57C polymorphisms were observed only in golden retrievers. The G246A and C660G polymorphisms were not observed in Maltese or miniature schnauzers in which the C allele of the G1146C and T955C polymorphisms was dominant, whereas other alleles were dominant in the other four breeds.

Ogata et al. (2006) identified a single nucleotide polymorphism (T199C) located on the putative third exon of the canine monoamine oxidase B gene, which causes an amino acid substitution from cysteine to arginine. They examined the allelic frequencies in five dog breeds (Golden retriever, Labrador retriever, Maltese, miniature schnauzer, and Shiba) and found significant variation among them.

Takeuchi et al. (2005) used brain cDNAs derived from ten unrelated Beagles to search for polymorphisms in tyrosine hydroxylase (TH) and dopamine beta hydroxylase (DBH), the enzymes synthesizing norepinephrine and dopamine, respectively. Four single nucleotide polymorphisms (SNPs) (C97T, G168A, G180A and C264T), one of which (C97T) will cause amino acid substitution in the TH gene, and two SNPs (C789A and A1819G), both of which will cause amino acid substitutions in the DBH gene were identified.

The allelic frequencies among five dog breeds (47 golden retrievers, 41 Labrador retrievers, 40 Malteses, 26 miniature schnauzers, and 39 Shibas) were examined and found to have significant variation between them with regards to all these SNPs, except for C97T in the TH gene and A181 9G in the DBH gene which were found only in the Shiba.

The alleles of 168A and 264T on the TH gene are found in relatively high frequency in the Labrador retrievers which are higher in ease of housebreaking and low on attention demand and general activity than the other breeds. At G180A, the Labrador retriever and miniature schnauzer, which rank higher in territorial defense, have more A alleles than the other breeds. At C789A, the ratio of allelic frequency of the golden and Labrador retrievers to other breeds is reversed. Retrievers rank lower in dominance over the owner, watch dog barking, snapping at children, destructiveness, aggression to other dogs, and excessive barking in comparison to other breeds.

Ogata et al. (2006) screened four excitatory amino acid transporters (EAAT) genes (glutamate transporter-1; GLT-1, excitatory amino acid transporter 4; EAAT4, excitatory amino acid carrier; EAAC1, glutamate/aspartate transporter; GLAST) for single nucleotide polymorphisms (SNPs). They identified two silent SNPs (C129T and T471C) in the GLT-1 gene. Next, they genotyped 193 dogs of 5 breeds and found significant variation among breeds in these two SNPs in GLT-1. The C129T polymorphism was not observed in Malteses and miniature schnauzers. The T allele variant of the C129T polymorphism was observed only in golden retrievers, Labradors and Shibas, breeds that have low excitability. Golden retrievers and Labradors had a relatively higher proportion of the C allele of the T471C polymorphism, the miniature schnauzers and Shiba had a higher proportion of the C and T allele; the C and T alleles were approximately equal in Maltese. Labrador retrievers and golden retrievers differ behaviorally from Shiba and schnauzers on defensive aggression.

11

Genetic Manipulation in Mouse

With the deciphering of the human genome, a major challenge is to determine the function for each of the estimated 30,000 genes in the physiology and patho-physiology of various organs. Using the mouse as a model system, this has been achieved by new genetic tools that restrict gene manipulation in a regional- and time-specific manner, thus bypassing the lethality caused by the traditional gene targeting approach, which inactivates gene function in the whole body and/or during embryogenesis. The major systems for regional and temporal gene manipulation include *site-specific recombinase* (SSR) systems and inducible transcription systems. Among these, the Cre-*lox*P SSR system, the Flp recombinase target (FRT) SSR system and the tetracycline (tet) regulatory systems are the most extensively used. Since the Cre-*lox*P and Flp-FRT system are quite similar in principle and methodology, in this chapter we will focus on the Cre-*lox*P, as well as the tet regulatory, system and describe their principles, applications, methodology and troubleshooting.

Cre-*lox*P System

Principles

The Cre-*lox*P system utilizes Cre-mediated DNA recombination. Cre, a site-specific recombinase derived from P1 phage, binds its 34 bp recognition site *lox*P and catalyzes a recombination event between two *lox*P sites. When two *lox*P sites of the same orientation are placed at the two ends of a DNA segment (i.e., the DNA segment is "floxed"),

Cre-mediated recombination would excise the DNA segment between the two *lox*P sites. By contrast, when two *lox*P sites of opposite orientation are placed at the two ends of a DNA segment, inversion of the floxed DNA segment will occur. To apply this system to mice, two transgenic mouse lines usually need to be generated: one with *Cre* driven by a region- or cell type-specific promoter, and another in which a segment of a target gene is floxed by two *lox*P sites of the same orientation (referred to hereafter as "*floxed* line"). In the doubly mutant mice, the target gene segment is deleted specifically in Cre-expressing regions and cell types. To completely inactivate the target gene in Cre-expressing areas, the floxed mice must be either homozygous or heterozygous (over a null allele, – that is to say one allele is deleted by traditional gene targeting, and the other allele is flanked by *lox*P sites), for the floxed gene. This system is also called

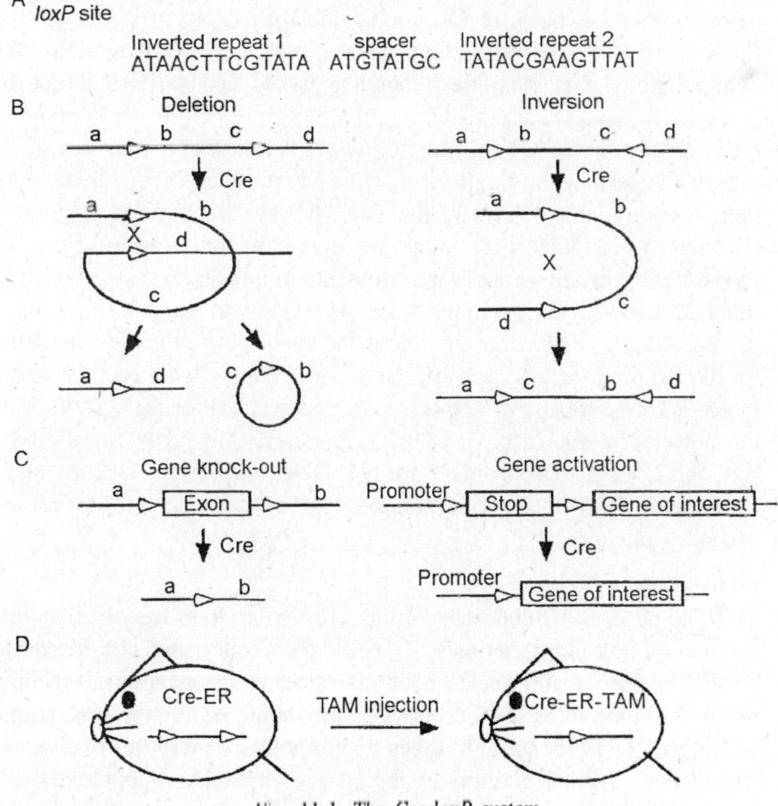

Fig. 11.1. The Cre-loxP system.

the "Cre-*lox*P conditional knock-out" system. Conversely, a "Cre-*lox*P conditional activation" system has been developed in which the *floxed* line harbors a *gene of interest* (GOI) driven by a constitutively active promoter but silenced transcriptionally and translationally due to a floxed STOP cassette [containing an array of SV40 polyadenylation (polyA) sequences and several translational stop codons in all reading frames] inserted between the GOI and its promoter.

Applications

Firstly, the Cre-*lox*P system has been a powerful tool for the study of gene function via conditional knock-out/activation. The recent development of mouse lines with ligand-inducible forms of Cre further offers the opportunity to temporally control Cre activity and subsequent gene manipulation at a later time following the onset of Cre expression. Secondly, the Cre-*lox*P system has become a popular tool for cell fate mapping studies, because Cre-mediated DNA excision is irreversible [in contrast to the tet regulatory system, which allows reversible gene manipulation]. For example, when the *floxed* line harbors a reporter [such as β-galactosidase (β-Gal), alkaline phosphatase (AP) or *green fluorescent protein* (GFP), etc] following a floxed STOP cassette, the reporter is permanently expressed in Cre-expressing cells and, notably, their progeny cells. Thirdly, the Cre-*lox*P system is being applied to chromosome engineering, including inversion and translocation, for modeling of chromosomal rearrangements in human diseases. Fourthly, mutated loxP sequences have been developed to elicit Cre-mediated recombination events that are independent of recombination mediated by the original (wild-type) loxP sequence. This allows recombination to occur between pairs of homotypic (e.g., *lox*P/*lox*P or *lox5171*/*lox5171*) but not heterotypic (e.g., *lox*P/*lox5171*) sites, thus providing the basis for stable exchange or inversion of DNA segments. Due to space limitations, we will describe methodology related only to the first and second applications.

Generating Cre Lines

The general methodology of the Cre-*lox*P system has been covered by several excellent reviews. General techniques and considerations for production of transgenic/knock-out mice, mouse handling, breeding, and genotyping have been described elsewhere. As for the time frame, cloning of DNA constructs takes 1–3 months, generation of *Cre* and *floxed* lines takes 1 month (in the case of transgenic approach) or 6 months (in the case of knock-in approach), and founder screening takes

3–6 months. Therefore, the analysis of doubly mutant mice usually starts at 6–12 months following the onset of the project.

A list of most, if not all, available *Cre* lines with corresponding reference and contact information is constantly updated in the Cre transgenic database on the Nagy group website. A new *Cre* line can be generated through either a transgenic or a knock-in approach. In the transgenic approach, the DNA construct consists of the *Cre* coding sequence sandwiched between a promoter and an intron/polyA sequence. (The choice of promoter depends on which region and cell type you wish to manipulate.) The *Cre* sequence is fused to a *nuclear localization signal* (NLS), to localize Cre in the nucleus and maximize Cre activity. The intron/polyA sequence, e.g., the SV40 intron/polyA fragment [*Xho*I/*Bam*HI-digested product of pMSG], is used to promote NLS-Cre expression. After the completion of cloning, the DNA construct is purified, linearized and injected into the pronuclei of fertilized eggs to obtain transgenic founders. In some cases, a gene that is expressed in a desired region and cell type has been identified, but its promoter has not been defined. In this case, a *bacterial artificial chromosome* (BAC) clone that contains the genomic sequence of the putative promoter can be used. If the BAC clone also carries the gene's translational initiation codon, *NLS-Cre* is recombined into the BAC clone, replacing the translational initiation codon, and the *NLS-Cre*-containing BAC is then injected into fertilized eggs. If the BAC clone does not carry the gene's translational initiation codon, the BAC clone can be coinjected into eggs with a DNA construct carrying *NLS-Cre* driven by a minimal promoter. When the BAC clone and the minimal promoter-*NLS-Cre* construct cointegrate into the chromosome, NLS-Cre would be expressed in the region and cell type defined by the BAC clone. To make a *Cre* line using a knock-in approach, *NLS-Cre* is recombined into a desired gene locus in embryonic stem (ES) cells, which are then injected into blastocysts to obtain chimeric founders.

Genotyping *Cre* Lines

Cre lines are genotyped by the presence of *Cre*. We use the following primers and PCR conditions: 5'-ACCTGATGGACATGTTCA GGGATCG-3' and 5'-TCCGGTTATTCAACTTGCACCATGC-3'; 94°C for 2 min, 30 cycles of 94°C for 50 s, 60°C for 1 min, 72°C for 1 min, then 72°C for 7 min. However, when different *Cre* lines need to be identified by genotyping, we would design one oligonucleotide in the 3' region of the promoter and the other complementary to the 5' region of *Cre*.

Screening *Cre* Lines

After confirmation of *Cre* by PCR and Southern blot analysis, positive founders are screened initially by their Cre expression level, first by immunohistochemistry and then by crossing with Cre-responsive reporter lines, to determine in which region and cell lineage recombination occurs. The reporter assay directly assesses the efficiency of Cre-mediated recombination, thus providing a more faithful indicator of Cre activity than Cre expression analysis. It should be cautioned, however, that the reporter assay may not predict the efficiency of the recombination event of a GOI in a specific *floxed* line, because the recombination efficiency could vary due to the chromosomal locus of the floxed allele and the distance between two loxP sites. Thus, one should determine the frequency and kinetics of target gene activation/inactivation with the specific *Cre* line and *floxed* line to be used for phenotypic analysis.

The most popular reporter lines are *R26R* and *Z/AP* mice. In R26R mice, β-*Gal*, together with an upstream floxed STOP cassette, is knocked into a constitutively and ubiquitously active locus *Rosa 26*. In doubly mutant mice *Cre;R26R*, β-Gal is expressed in regions and cell lineages where the *STOP* cassette is deleted by Cre-mediated recombination. In *Z/AP* mice, *AP*, driven by the CAG promoter (chicken β-actin promoter coupled with cytomegalovirus enhancer), is silenced by a floxed *STOP* cassette that contains the β-*Gal* sequence. In doubly mutant mice *Cre;Z/AP*, β-Gal is expressed in regions and cell lineages without Cre-mediated recombination, whereas AP is expressed in regions and cell lineages with Cre-mediated recombination. This double reporter system thus provides a convenient and reliable indicator of Cre activity. Protocols to detect Cre, β-Gal and AP are described below. When GFP and other color variant fluorescent proteins are used as reporters, the whole embryo/tissue or sections of animal/tissue can be directly examined under a fluorescence microscope.

Immunohistochemistry for Cre

For Cre staining in tissue sections, the mice are perfused with cold saline (0.9% NaCl) for 10 min, and cold 4% paraformaldehyde (PFA)/phosphate-buffered saline (PBS) for 30 min and the tissue dissected out and post-fixed in the same fixative at 4°C overnight. On the following day, the tissue is sectioned in cold PBS at 50 μm thickness by a Vibratome. Sections can then be stored in PBS at 4°C for up to 6 months, until use. Sections are blocked in 5% goat serum/0.2% Triton X-100/PBS at room temperature for 1.5 h, and incubated with a rabbit anti-Cre antibody at 1:2,000–3,000 dilution in 1% goat serum/0.1% Triton X-100/PBS, with gentle shaking at 4°C overnight. After washing three times with PBS (each for 10 min), sections are incubated with appropriately diluted secondary antibody [e.g., Alexa 488-conjugated anti-rabbit IgG at 1:300 dilution] in 1% goat serum/0.1% Triton X-100/PBS, at room temperature for 1.5 h. After washing three times with PBS, (each for 10 min), sections are mounted onto slides by floating in PBS, then air-dried and overlaid with coverslips under Vectashield mounting medium. To localize Cre expression, sections can be double-stained with anti-Cre antibody and an antibody that is produced from a species other than rabbit.

Immunohistochemistry for β-Gal

β-Gal staining follows the same procedures as Cre staining above, except that a rabbit anti-β-gal antibody, at 1:2,000 dilution, is used as the primary antibody.

X-Gal staining

For whole-mount X-gal staining of embryos and tissues, small embryos and tissues are rinsed in PBS followed by fixation with X-gal fixative (PBS containing 1% formaldehyde, 0.2% glutaraldehyde, 2 mM $MgCl_2$, 5 mM EGTA and 0.02% NP-40), with gentle shaking at 4°C for 30–60 min. Larger embryos (E13.5 or older) or tissues are fixed in the same fixative at 4°C for 60–90 min. Following fixation, samples are washed three times (each for 5–10 min) in PBS/0.02% NP-40 and incubated in X-gal staining buffer (PBS containing 1 mg=ml X-gal, 5 mM potassium ferrocyanide, 5 mM potassium ferricyanide, 2 mM $MgCl_2$, 0.01% sodium deoxycholate and 0.02% NP-40), at 37°C for 30 min to 24 h. (Note that samples should be protected from light during the X-gal reaction). After completion of staining, samples are washed three times (each for 5 min) in PBS, post-fixed in PBS/4% PFA and stored in PBS/80% glycerol, at 4°C, or photographed. It should be noted that the penetration of X-gal becomes much weaker in embryos or tissues of larger size, thus we recommend performing X-gal staining on frozen sections. Larger embryos and embryonic tissues are fixed following the above procedure. For adult tissues, mice are perfused with cold PBS/4% PFA for 15–30 min. The desired tissue is dissected out and post-fixed in the same fixative at 4°C for 1–2 h. After fixation, samples are washed in PBS three times (each for 5–10 min), cryoprotected in PBS/30% sucrose at 4°C overnight, incubated in OCT medium at room temperature for 30 min and transferred to –20°C overnight. Sections are cut at 10 μm thickness with a Cryostat, placed onto polylysine-coated or ProbeOn Plus slides, air dried for 30 min and then, if necessary, stored at -20°C for 1–2 months until use. On the day of staining, sections are taken out to room temperature for 10–15 min, washed three times with X-gal wash buffer, (X-gal staining buffer without X-gal, each for 10 min), and incubated in X-gal staining buffer at 37°C, for 30 min to 24 h (light protected). After completion of staining, sections can be counterstained with nuclear staining reagents such as Nuclear Fast Red, rinsed in PBS, dehydrated through a graded ethanol series and xylene, and mounted with Permount. The percentage of X-gal-positive neurons out of the total number of neurons (identified by Fast Red-positive) indicates the frequency of Cre-*lox*P recombination.

X-gal and AP double-staining

For whole-mount double-staining, samples are fixed similarly as for the X-gal staining protocol above, except that 0.01% sodium deoxycholate is added to X-gal fixative to allow better penetration of AP substrates. After processing with X-gal staining, samples are rinsed in PBS, incubated in PBS at 70–75°C for 30 min to remove endogenous AP, rinsed again in PBS, washed in AP buffer, (100 mM Tris-HCl pH 9.5, 100 mM NaCl and 10 mM $MgCl_2$), for 10 min and stained with BM Purple AP substrate at 4°C for 0.5–24 h. After completion of staining, samples are washed extensively with PBS/0.1% Tween-20/2 mM $MgCl_2$. For double-staining of frozen sections, sections are fixed and X-gal stained and then washed in PBS three times (each for 5 min), incubated in PBS at 70–75°C for 30 min, rinsed again in PBS, washed in AP buffer for 10 min, and overlaid with NBT/BCIP staining buffer [100 mM Tris-HCl pH 9.5, 100 mM NaCl and 50 mM $MgCl_2$, 0.01% sodium deoxycholate, 0.02% NP-40, 337 μg/ml nitroblue tetrazolium salt and 175 μg/ml 5-bromo-4-chloro-3-indolyl phosphate, toluidinium salt (BCIP)] at room temperature for 10–30 min. After completion of staining, sections are rinsed in PBS, dehydrated through a graded ethanol series and mounted. The staining signal (X-gal in blue and AP in dark red) is visualized and photographed under a light microscope.

Generating Floxed Lines

Conditional knock-outs

LoxP sites are usually inserted into the introns of a target gene to preserve the gene's expression. A conditional targeting replacement construct consists of a 5'-flanking region, *loxP* site 1, the intron/exon region to be deleted, *loxP* site 2, *LFNT* cassette, a 3'-flanking region and *diphtheria toxin* (*DT-A*). The LFNT cassette consists of a second pair of loxP sites, a pair of FRT sites, and pgk-*neo* and hsv-*tk* selection markers. Thus, recombined ES clones are initially selected for the presence of a *neo* marker, then transfected with Flp or Cre to remove the LFNT cassette and selected for the absence of a *tk* marker. DT-A provides an additional marker to select against non-homologous recombinants. In addition to constructing such targeting vectors via classical cloning methods, recent advancement in BAC technology provides a new and rapid means to insert loxP sites directly into ES cells. In both cases, the resulting ES clones are injected into blastocysts, and chimeric, germline transmitting founders are confirmed by Southern blot analysis of tissue from offspring. By crossing the *floxed* line to a desired *Cre* line, the kinetics and location of target gene removal are monitored by RNA in situ hybridization and immuno-histochemistry, as described below.

Conditional activation

In a conditional activation construct, a GOI, together with an upstream floxed STOP cassette, is inserted between a constitutively active promoter and an intron/polyA sequence. The GOI can be a wild-type, constitutively active, or dominant/negative form of a gene. When the GOI is a dominant/negative form, it should be functionally potent (considering the much lower number of copies expressed in transgenic or knock-in mice than in transfected cells), and highly specific to the gene to be manipulated, in order to avoid potential quenching of its binding partners. The GOI is monitored by epitope-tagging with a myc, flag, hemagglutinin (HA), or GFP tag. The *floxed* line can be generated through either a transgenic or knock-in approach, following procedures similar to those used in the generation of *Cre* lines above. Once founders are obtained, they are screened by crossing with a desired *Cre* line to determine the level of Cre-mediated expression of the GOI. (Note that a good founder line should also possess very low levels of GOI expression in the absence of Cre). In doubly mutant mice, the level of GOI expression is determined by either RNA in situ hybridization and/or immunohistochemistry, as described below.

RNA in situ Hybridization

Note that all reagents and equipment must be RNase-free [e.g., RNase-free Eppendorf tubes from Marsh], and PBS and water must be pretreated with diethyl pyrocarbonate (DEPC).

Probe preparation

^{33}P-Labeled RNA probes are prepared via in vitro transcription from a DNA template consisting of a promoter (T7, T3 or SP6) and the probe region (300–500 bases long) and terminating at the end of the probe region (so the RNA polymerase will fall off the template). The DNA template can be generated by PCR using a pair of primers, each of which includes a T7, T3 or SP6 promoter sequence plus one of the two ends of the probe region. Alternatively, the probe region can be cloned into a vector containing the T7, T3 or SP6 promoter (e.g., pSP72), which is then cut at one end of the probe region by a restriction enzyme. After purification, the DNA template is subjected to in vitro transcription using a ribo-probe system T7, T3 or SP6 kit (Promega) following the manufacturer's instructions. For ^{33}P-UTP, we use EasyTides uridine 5'-triphosphate- [α-^{33} P]. To remove the DNA template, the in vitro transcription reaction mix (15 μl) is incubated with 6 μl DNase mix (including 1 μl RNasin, 4 μl tRNA at 5 μg/ml and 1 μl RQ1 DNase) at 37°C for 15 min. The unincorporated ^{33}P-UTP is further removed by use of a spin column. Next, to determine the amount of ^{33}P-UTP incorporation, the purified probe is diluted 1:500 in TE buffer, of which 5 μl is transferred to 4 ml water-soluble liquid scintillator and counted in a liquid scintillation counter, using the ^{14}C, ^{32}S and ^{33}P range. The count must be at least 3,000 cpm, and ideally around 8,000 cpm. If the count is lower than 3,000 cpm, repeat the procedure by making new DNA template and/or new probe by adding more template.

Pretreatment of tissue sections

Tissues should be rapidly dissected from anaesthetized mice, placed into Peel-a-way embedding molds (VWR), and covered with OCT medium. Embedded tissues are frozen at –20°C overnight for immediate use, or stored at –80°C for use within 6 months. (In the latter case, tissues should be transferred back to –20°C the night before cutting). After equilibration at –20°C, tissues are cut at 14 μm thickness with a cryostat, and sections are mounted onto ProbeOn Plus slides. Mounted sections can be stored at –80°C for up to 6 months. On the day of hybridization, sections are left at room temperature for 30 min, stacked on a slide holder and processed using a Tissue-Tek slide staining set (VWR). Sections are fixed with 4% PFA/PBS for 20 min, treated with 10 μg/ml proteinase K in 10 mM Tris-HCl pH 8.0/1 mM EDTA at 37°C for 30 min, post-fixed with 4% PFA/PBS for 15 min, rinsed with PBS for 2 min, and treated with 0.2 M HCl for 10 min. Note that too much active proteinase K can generate holes in sections. Therefore, one should determine the appropriate concentration for proteinase K for each batch purchased. After rinsing with PBS and 0.1 M triethanolamine (TEA), sections are further incubated in 0.25% acetic anhydride/0.1 M TEA, for 10 min, to avoid non-specific binding of the probe. Following dehydration through a graded ethanol series (70% to 80% to 90% to 100%) and chloroform, sections are air-dried for 30 min.

Hybridization

Hybridization buffer [50% formamide, 10 mM Tris-HCl pH 8, 200 μg/ml tRNA (RNase-free), 1X Denhardt's solution, 10% dextran sulfate, 600 mM NaCl, 0.25% SDS and 1 mM EDTA pH 8; stored at 4°C], is preheated to 85°C for 10 min. The probe is diluted 1:20 in this preheated hybridization buffer, then heated at 85°C for 5 min followed by abrupt chill in icy water for over 5 min (to maintain the probe in an open conformation). The sections are then covered with the diluted probe at 150 μl per slide ($\sim 1.2 \times 10^8$ cpm) and overlaid with a picce of Parafilm precut to the size of the slide. (Bubbles should be avoided to prevent areas of non-hybridization). The slides are then placed on several layers of Whatman paper, previously wet by 50% formamide, in a box and placed within a 55°C incubator overnight.

Washing and exposure

After the Parafilm is removed, sections are washed at 55°C with 5X SSC for 30 min and 50% formamide/2X SSC for 30 min. At 37°C, sections are then washed with TNE (10 mM Tris-HCl pH 7.6, 500 mM NaCl and 1 mM EDTA) for 10 min, treated in 12.5 μg/ml RNase A/TNE for 30 min and washed with TNE for 10 min. Next, at 55°C, sections are washed with 2X SSC twice (each for 30 min) and 0.2X SSC twice (each for 30 min), followed by dehydration through a graded ethanol series (70% to 80% to 90% to 95%) in 0.3 M ammonium acetate and 100% ethanol, and air dried. The slides are exposed to BioMax MR film and developed in a darkroom.

Dipping and development of micro-autoradiography

To visualize hybridization signals at a higher resolution, the slides are dipped three times in NTB3 nuclear emulsion diluted with glycerol (1:1). Note that the entire dipping process must be performed in the dark or under red light. After immersion, the emulsion solution on the back side of the slide is wiped away with a Kimwipe paper. The slide is air dried for 1 h, transferred to a slide box with silica gel and stored at 4°C in the dark for 4–8 weeks. To develop micro-autoradiography, the slides are incubated in D-19 solution for 5 min, dipped in water several times, incubated in F-5 solution for 5 min, extensively washed by flowing water for 15 min and air dried. The hybridization signals should appear as black dots under a light microscope. To determine which cell type and subcellular compartment shows a positive hybridization signal, the sections can be further stained with Nissl and other counter-stains.

Tyramide Signal Amplification (TSA) for Fluorescence Immunostaining

Regular immunofluorescence staining by incubating tissue sections with primary and secondary antibodies can be carried out following the protocol described above for Cre and β-Gal staining. To enhance detection sensitivity, we utilize the TSA system (NEN), which uses horseradish peroxidase to catalyze the deposition of biotin-labeled tyramide (amplification reagent) onto tissue sections. By following the manufacturer's instructions, we find that this system shows high sensitivity and low background in signal detection. If the primary antibody is generated from mouse, we usually use the MOM kit (Vector) together with the TSA system, to avoid nonspecific staining of mouse IgG.

Temporally Controllable Cre-loxP System

Ligand-inducible forms of Cre have been developed by fusing a mutant *estrogen receptor* (ER) ligand-binding domain to the carboxyl terminus of Cre. Cre-ER is sequestered in the cytoplasm by Hsp90 and remains inactive until it binds to synthetic estrogen agonist 4-OH-tamoxifen (4-OH-TAM), which disrupts the interaction between Cre-ER and Hsp90. Note that TAM, which is converted to its active derivative 4-OH-TAM in the liver, is often administered in preference to 4-OH-TAM, because TAM is more soluble in solvents like corn oil. Using various promoters to drive Cre-ER expression, several *Cre-ER* mouse lines have shown promising potential to add temporal control to the Cre-*loxP* system. For instance, using the ubiquitously active CAG promoter, Cre-ER-mediated recombination was seen to be detectable in many tissues and cell types by 15 h post TAM injection, and peaked by 48 h. Thus, new *Cre-ER* lines that express *Cre-ER* (one of three forms: *Cre-ER*^{TM}, *Cre-ER*^{T} and *Cre-ER*^{T2}) in a desired region and cell type can be generated with protocols similar to those described above. After crossing a *Cre-ER* line to a Cre-responsive reporter line (preferably a double-reporter line, like *Z/AP*), one can determine the efficiency of recombination in a desired tissue or cell type by X-gal/AP staining and/or immunohistochemistry. An optimal degree of recombination is determined by the injection of increasing doses of TAM, up to the point at which toxicity becomes apparent (e.g., 6–8 mg for a 30 g animal, and 9 mg mg for an animal of 40 g or more). TAM is dissolved in corn oil at up to 20 mg/ml at 65°C with gentle stirring and can be stored at 4°C for 3–4 weeks, until a white precipitate appears. When a *Cre-ER* line is crossed to a *floxed* line in conditional knock-out/activation experiments, RNA in situ hybridization and/or immunohistochemistry should be performed to determine the degree of Cre-ER-mediated recombination.

Tetracycline Regulatory System

Principles

The tet regulatory system regulates gene expression at the transcriptional level via a tet-controlled transcriptional activator (tTA). tTA is a fusion product of the repressor of *Escherichia coli Tn10* tet-resistant operon and the carboxyl-terminal portion of herpes simplex virus protein VP16 that functions as a strong transcriptional activator. The GOI is driven by an array of tet operator (*tetO*) sequences, followed by a minimal promoter (*Pmin*). In the absence of tet, tTA binds to *tetO* and activates GOI transcription, whereas in the presence of tet, tTA is sequestered by tet from *tetO* and GOI transcription is inactivated. To apply this system to mice, two mouse lines usually need to be generated: one with tTA driven by a region-, or cell-type-specific, promoter (hereafter referred to as "tTA regulator line"), and the other with a GOI driven by *tetO-Pmin* (hereafter referred to as "tet responsive line"). In doubly mutant mice, GOI transcription will be active – only in the region or cells defined by the promoter upstream of *tTA* – in the absence of tet but inactive in the presence of tet. Thus, this system is also called the "tet-off" system. Conversely, the "tet-on" system has been developed via the generation of a mutant form of tTA, reverse tet-controlled transactivator (rtTA), which activates gene transcription only in the presence of tet.

Applications

By temporally expressing a wild-type, constitutively active, or dominant/ negative form of a GOI, the tet regulatory system is used to study gene function within a desired time period, e.g., in adulthood, following the completion of development. The reversibility of gene

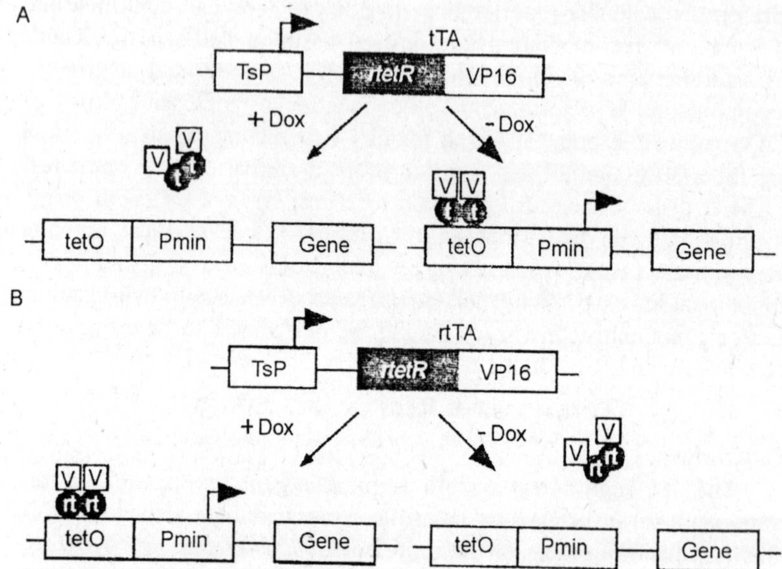

Fig. 11.2. The tetracycline (tet) regulatory system.

manipulation further allows identification of critical time periods for gene function. Thus, by temporally manipulating disease-related genes, in recent years this system has become an invaluable tool for modeling the cause and progression of human diseases in mice. After the appearance of disease-like symptoms, expression of these genes can be turned off to further assess the consequence of their elimination. This is instrumental in the development of therapeutic strategies.

Generating tTA/rtTA Regulator Lines

The methodology of the tTA and rtTA systems is largely interchangeable. However, it should be noted that the tTA and rtTA systems differ not only in their opposite dependency on tet, or its more potent derivative doxycycline (dox), for transactivation, but also in their kinetics of transactivation/inactivation. In the tTA system, silencing of the GOI upon dox treatment was achieved in embryos after 6 h and in adults after 5 days. Conversely, expression of a GOI upon dox withdrawal depends on the rate of dox clearance and could take from 24 h to 1 week. By contrast, in the rtTA system, expression of a GOI upon dox treatment was achieved in embryos within 13 h and in adults within 1 h. Thus, one should examine the kinetics of gene activation/inactivation with the specific combination of tTA/rtTA regulator and tet responsive lines to be used for phenotypic analysis.

In the adult brain, full rtTA-dependent activation of gene expression is achieved only by supplying dox at up to 10 mg/g food, due to the limited ability of dox to penetrate the *blood brain barrier* (BBB). Therefore, despite a few reports, the rtTA system has not been used as extensively as the tTA system to study brain function. To overcome this, an rtTA variant with a higher dox-sensitivity or a dox variant with higher penetration of the BBB must be developed. Regarding the time frame for analysis, as with the Cre-*loxP* system, analysis of doubly mutant mice in the tet regulatory system usually starts at 6–12 months following the onset of the project.

A list of most, if not all, available tTA/rtTA regulator lines, with corresponding references and contact information, is available at the website. A new tTA/rtTA regulator line can be generated through either a transgenic or knock-in approach, similar to the methods described above for generating *Cre* lines. *tTA* can be subcloned from plasmid pUHD15–1 and *rtTA* from plasmid pUHG17–1. Both of these plasmids, together with data sheets, can be obtained from the laboratory. Alternatively, similar plasmids can be purchased from Clontech.

Genotyping tTA/rtTA Regulator Lines

The tTA/rtTA regulator lines are genotyped by identifying the presence of tTA/rtTA. Since rtTA differs from tTA by only four amino acids, the same primers can usually be used to genotype either tTA or rtTA regulator lines. For instance, we use primers 5'ATAAGCGGG CTTTGCTCGAC3' and 5'taagaaggCTGGCTCTGCAC3' and our PCR conditions are: 94°C for 2 min, 30 cycles of 94°C for 50 s, 60°C for 1 min, 72°C for 1 min, followed by 72°C for 7 min.

Screening tTA/rtTA Regulator Lines

After confirmation of *tTA/rtTA* by PCR and Southern blot analysis, positive founder animals are screened by crossing with tet responsive reporter lines. In doubly mutant mice, the level of reporter expression is monitored both in the absence and in the presence of dox. The Bujard laboratory routinely dissolves dox-HCl (Sigma) in 5% sucrose at a final concentration of 200 μg/ml. The water bottle should be light protected and the dox-containing water should be renewed every 3 days. Alternatively, dox-containing food pellets are available at multiple concentrations (20 mg/kg–6 g/kg) and can be obtained at a specific concentration by custom order. To test tet-regulated reporter expression in doubly mutant mice, we start at 1 week following feeding with dox water at 200 μg/ml or dox diet at 200 mg/kg. Depending on the result, we then alter the feeding agenda by lengthening/shortening the feeding period and/or increasing/decreasing dox concentration. When used at these doses, doxycycline is not toxic. However, if it is necessary to give very high doses of doxycycline to control the transgene, the drug will accumulate in the tissues of the animal. Thus, it will take a long time for the animal to eliminate the accumulated drug from its body before the transgene can be regulated again. For a good tTA regulator line, reporter expression should be robust in the absence of tet and quickly turned off upon dox treatment. Conversely, for a good rtTA regulator line, reporter expression should be silent (or very low) in the absence of tet, and quickly rise and reach robust levels upon dox treatment.

The most popular reporter lines are *tetO-β-gal* and *tetO-GFP*, because they allow the identification of the region and cell type within which the transgene is turned on/off. In the *tetO-GFP* system, embryos/ tissues or sections of embryo/tissue from the doubly mutant mice are directly examined under a fluorescence microscope. In the *tetO-β-gal* system, mice are subjected to X-gal staining or β-gal immunohistochemistry.

Generating tet-Responsive Lines

Tet-responsive lines are usually generated by pronuclear injection of a DNA construct consisting of a GOI sandwiched between *tetO-Pmin* and an intron/polyA sequence. The GOI is monitored either by epitope-tagging or by placing it under the control of a bidirectional *tetO-Pmin*. Via tTA/rtTA and dox, the bidirectional *tetO-Pmin* co-regulates transcription of two genes in opposite directions. This enables the simultaneous transcriptional activation/inactivation of GOI and a reporter gene, such as β-gal, luciferase or GFP. Cloning vectors for both uni- and bi-directional tet-responsive lines, with data sheets, can be obtained from the Bujard laboratory.

Genotyping tet-Responsive Lines

We design one primer in the *tetO* sequence (e.g., 5'TGAAAGTC GAGCTCGGTACC3') and the other complementary to part of *Pmin* or GOI. The primers are generally 20–21 bases long with 50–55% G+C and terminate with a C or G. The PCR conditions are the same as those used for genotyping tTA/rtTA regulator lines.

Screening tet-Responsive Lines

Due to the variability in transgene integration site and the number of integrated copies, tet-responsive lines can exhibit various levels of basal expression (in the absence of tTA/rtTA and dox) and tTA/rtTA-dependent expression. Basal expression is tested in founder mice or their progeny in the absence of tTA/rtTA and dox, while tTA/rtTA-dependent expression is tested by crossing the founder to a desired tTA/rtTA line. In these doubly mutant mice, tet regulation is further tested by varying the dose and length of dox treatment. A good tet-responsive line should exhibit a low level of basal expression, and a robust level of expression in the presence of tTA or rtTA plus dox, which is tightly regulated by dox. To monitor GOI expression, we use RNA in situ hybridization or immunohistochemistry, both of which allow the identification of regions of gene expression. As with the bi-directional tet responsive lines, it is important to verify, by in situ hybridization of consecutive sections, or by performing double immunostaining using antibodies raised against the GOI and reporter, that the GOI and the reporter do express in the same region and in the same cell types.

In the tTA system, GOI can be kept silent by dox treatment and then turned on by dox withdrawal. It should be cautioned that turning on of gene expression of GOI following dox withdrawal may not be quick, and expression may not reach the same level as in mice that have never been subjected to dox treatment. This, in our experience, occurs particularly when dox is administered during the gestation period to the pregnant mother, presumably due to incorporation of dox into bones and other tissues and consequent alteration in chromatin structure during embryogenesis. Thus, it is important firstly to determine and then to apply the lowest dose of dox in order to shut off gene expression in one's own doubly mutant mice and with one's own lab setup.

New Directions for Regional and Temporal Gene Manipulation

Firstly, quantitative control of gene activity can be achieved by varying the TAM dose in a Cre-ER-*loxP* system, or dox dose in a tet regulatory system. With a means to identify cells that have undergone gene activation/inactivation, the properties of these cells can be investigated and compared with wild-type neighbors. This would provide an efficient way to dissect the roles of gene function through cell-cell interactions. Secondly, inducible and reversible gene inactivation can be achieved by tet-regulated expression of a GOI in mice with a null or conditional null mutation of this gene. Temporal restoration of gene function in a desired region and cell type will provide a versatile tool for determination of the critical period and area of gene function. In order to overcome the time and expense involved in intercrossing multiple lines, (e.g., tTA/rtTA regulatory line, tet responsive line, knockout line), several groups have developed an elegant strategy for the insertion of a regulatory cassette (containing a STOP cassette and *tetO-Pmin*) into the 5'-UTR region of a GOI, such that transcription of this endogenous gene becomes regulated by tTA/rtTA. Thirdly, the combination of tet regulatory and Cre-*loxP* systems will provide refined temporal control to region-specific gene manipulation, when Cre expression is regulated by tet. Alternatively, when tet and Cre-ER independently regulate the expression of two genes, these genes can be sequentially activated/inactivated by administration of dox and TAM, respectively. This would be advantageous in the modeling of human diseases such as cancer, where mutation in several genes occurs sequentially.

12

Alleles and Genotypes in Sheep

The study of the genetic structure within animal populations is of significant importance for the improvement of their selection with regard to higher productivity and enhanced resistance against infectious and parasitic diseases. For this purpose, various polymorphic systems are used (protein, erythrocyte, lymphocyte antigens, etc.). In humans, the polymorphism of C3 complement component has been fully studied. A relationship has been discovered between some C3 alleles and the susceptibility (or resistance) to some diseases. Very few reports about polymorphism of this factor in sheep currently exist. This situation consequently underlined our desire to carry out the present study with a view to determining the gene and genotype frequency of the polymorphic C3 system in the sheep.

Materials and Methods

Animals

The sheep included in this study were from 3 productive types:

A. *Milk type crossings*: 118 sheep and 14 rams - *Stara Zagora* × *East-Friesian* and (*Stara Zagora* × *East-Friesian*) × *Blackhead Pleven breeds*;

B. *Merino type*: 80 sheep and 9 rams from the *Trakia merino* breed;

C. *Meat type*: 107 sheep from the *Ile-de-France* breed and 107 sheep from the *Charollais* breed;

At the beginning of the experiment, the sheep and rams were aged between 2 and 3 years. They were housed in separate premises.

Blood for analysis was drawn from the *v. jugularis* and stored in 10 ml tubes. Subsequently, the blood was allowed to clot for one hour at room temperature (25°C) and the samples were finally centrifuged for 10 min. at 2000g.

Methods

The polymorphism of C3 complement component was determined according to the method of Teisberg described briefly as stated below:

Buffers

(a) Stock solutions for gels - 5,5-diethylbarbituric acid sodium salt 0.0230 M; 5,5-diethylbarbituric acid 0.0037 M; Calcium-L(+)-lactate 0.0009 M; pH=8.6.

(b) Stock solution for tray buffer – 5,5-diethylbarbituric acid sodium salt 0.061 M; 5,5-diethylbarbituric acid 0.01 M; Calcium- L(+)-lactate 0.00 18 M; pH=8.6.

1. The first buffer was used for preparation of agarose gel (1%) where serum samples were applied and electrophoresis carried out for about 2.5 h at 20 V/cm. Subsequently the gel was stained for 1 min with Amido Black 10 B and destained overnight with the destaining solution described below.
2. Destaining solution: ethanol, distilled water and glacial acetic acid (5:5:1) were mixed (for example, 1 l destaining solution contains 450 ml ethanol, 450 ml distilled water and 100 ml glacial acetic acid). Then 2 tablespoons of active charcoal powder were added in order to allow for the manifold use of the destaining solution.
3. Staining solution – 1% amido black 10B was added to 1 l destaining solution (without active charcoal ethanol), shaken well and left overnight. If necessary it could be filtered after a week.

The gene and genotype frequencies were calculated by the method of Nicholas, since it has been earlier established that the genes coding for the C3 complement component in sheep are inherited co-dominantly.

Results and Discussion

In our previous study, we had reported that the C3 complement component of the complement's system in sheep had a polymorphic structure; hence the frequency of the established alleles and genotypes could be calculated. For this purpose, we established the frequencies of the alleles S, F, F_1, and S_1, coding for the C3 complement component in the complement's system in sheep of three types – milk type, meat type (*Ile-de-France* and *Charollais*), and I type (*Trakia merino*). In the *Charollais* breed, the opposite phenomenon was observed as it had the F allele with a higher frequency. Typical of that breed was the appearance of another allele – F_1. Its frequency was low, yet it was present in the genetic structure of the studied population of the *Charollais* sheep. In the *Trakia merino* sheep, we observed a fourth allele – S_1. It also had a very low frequency – 0.04.

We determined that the four alleles described above formed nine genotypes – SS, FF, FS, F_7S, F_5S, $F_{10}S$, FF_1, SS_1, and S_1S_1. Their frequencies were different and depended on the breed; the most common was the homozygous genotype SS. Next was the heterozygous genotype FS that had the highest frequency in the *Charollais* breed. It was interesting to observe that the F_7S genotype had a very high frequency in two of the breeds (*Ile-de-France* – 0.33 and *Trakia merino* – 0.32).

Table 12.1. Relative frequencies of C3 gentypes in different sheep breeds

Genotypes	*Milk typecrossings*	*Il de France*	*Charolais*	*Trakia merino*
SS	0,36	0,36	0,18	0,25
FF	0,08	0,09	0,17	0,17
FS	0,34	0,22	0,20	0,20
F_7S	0,15	0,33	0,13	0,32
F_5S	0,07	-	0,14	-
$F_{10}S$	-	-	0,10	-
FF_1	-	-	0,08	-
SS_1	-	-	-	0,03
S_1S_1	-	-	-	0,03

As already stated, the C3 polymorphism in humans has been thoroughly studied. Wieme and Demeulenaere studied the polymorphism of human serum proteins and found that in some individuals, the β_2C globulin zone presented 2 bands in electrophoresis. The electrophoresis was performed in 1% agar gel but when the traditional starch gel was used the results were identical. Family analysis on these bands showed that they were inherited as an autosomal sign; but it did not indicate how. An interesting observation was the fact that the person with two β_2C bands was a girl suffering from the Hodgkin's disease. This first observation motivated the work of many investigators thereafter.

It was only one year later that Alper and Propp, using agarose gel with a better resolution, reported about 4 (probably 5) alleles, coding for C3 variants, and having different electrophoretic mobility.

They determined 15 various phenotypes. According to the authors, the F_1, F and S alleles were inherited co-dominantly in an autosomal fashion, whereas the S_1 and F0.8 alleles – via an unknown mechanism. Furthermore, the investigators studied the influence of various C3 genotypes on the blood serum C3 complement component concentration, the total complement activity and the adhesive properties of C3 molecules, but no significant differences had been observed.

The actual study on C3 polymorphism, however, began when Teisberg published a truly perfect method for C3 complement component electrophoresis in humans. The author reported that the frequency of the C3S allele was 0.80, and that of the C3F allele – 0.19. The following year Teisberg conducted a much broader research on Lapland people and discovered that the frequency of C3S was 0.9369, while C3F had a frequency of 0.0631.

The determined frequencies of those alleles in Norwegians were much different from those in Lapland people. In that same year, the researcher performed a new broad research that covered the whole territory of Norway (without Lapland) and discovered that the C3S allele had a frequency of 0.7865, while the frequency of C3F was 0.2082. Comparing those two values, he noticed a difference of 0.0053 that was created by the existence of seven very rare alleles ($C3F_{0.5}$; $C3F_{0.8}$; $C3F_{1.1}$; $C3S_{0.6}$; $C3S_{0.8}$; $C3S_{0.4}$; $C3S_{0.9}$). The totality of those nine alleles formed 13 different genotypes. The author was right to talk about genotypes because the mentioned alleles are inherited co-dominantly, as he personally found out.

Alper and Rosen summarised in a detailed overview that, besides the two common alleles (C3S and C3F), there were 14 other rare variants that have very low frequencies. They determined another very important fact – those versions were not different in terms of antigen and function. The molecular mechanism that leads to the polymorphism of the C3 complement component in humans was clarified by Botto et al. They determined that the difference between the genome organisation of C3S and C3F was a point mutation (cytosine to guanine) at nucleotide 364, exon 3. At a translation level, this resulted in replacement of arginine (at C3S) with glycine (at C3F). This replacement changes the polymorphous restriction area of the HhaI enzyme.

Using a genome DNA, RFLP was studied. Afterwards, the number of fragments was increased via PCR (polymerase chain reaction) and an absolute conformability between genome polymorphism and the distribution of C3S and C3F in 50 normal individuals was observed.

The molecular basis of the secondary structural polymorphism was determined via a HAV4-1 monoclonal antibody. The polymorphous determinate was established at codon 314 in exon 9 of the β-chain where leucine (HAV4-1^{+}) was replaced by proline (HAV4-1^{-}). The determination of amino acid sequences of those polymorphic variants would facilitate the characterisation of the probable functional differences among the various C3 allotypes.

The authors evidenced an increased incidence of the C3F allele in humans with partial lipodystrophy, IgA nephropathy, and Indian juvenile liver cirrhosis. Most probably, C3F could be used as a genetic marker for the determination of the susceptibility (or the resistance) to some diseases. In two studies, Dissing et al. and Sorensen and Dissing determined that the frequency of the C3F allele was higher in people suffering from arteriosclerosis. The relative risk of this disease was 1.87 times greater in C3F-positive individuals, in comparison with C3F-negative.

Bronestam and Cedergren reported a very interesting relationship between the high serum antibody titres and blood type antigens A and B in mothers that had recently given birth, and the carriers of the C3S allele. That phenomenon is observed very often in cases of ABO incompatibility between the mother and the infant. That fact leads to the idea that the carriers of the C3S gene would react with a higher immune response after vaccinations against infectious diseases. During the same year, Bronestam discovered a statistically feasible association between the C3F allele and the ratio of people affected by rheumatoid arthritis.

So far, the overview has shown that the polymorphism of the C3 complement component in humans has been studied thoroughly. Unfortunately, this problem has not been worked on sufficiently with animals. Gorman et al. reported the existence of C3 polymorphism in dogs. It was determined that C3F and C3S alleles were inherited co-dominantly in an autosomal fashion, but no other alleles were found. The locus of C3 is not linked and is inherited in accordance with neither the main histocompatibility complex genes (DLA) nor with the loci of C6 and C7 complement components.

The studies of Kay et al. in horses evidenced that in this animal species, the principal alleles were three: $C3_1$, $C3_2$ and $C3_3$, inherited co-dominantly as well. Those three alleles formed six various genotypes. Four years later, Bowling and Dileanis reported the existence of a fourth allele that was with a higher frequency only in the wild Prjevalsky horse and with very low frequencies (0.01-0.04) in three other breeds. Gahne and Amorena discovered a C3-like protein in sheep blood plasma. Unlike the earlier studies, they used an ordinary agarose gel electrophoresis followed by immunoblotting. Thus, they found 4 principal alleles, three of them (F, I, M) presenting one principal band and the fourth (S) –3 to 5 bands. The family analysis showed that the alleles were inherited co-dominantly in an autosomal manner. Until now, we have not found any information concerning the relationship between C3 polymorphism and resistance or susceptibility to diseases in animals.

13

GENE EXPRESSION ANALYSIS

Detailed analysis of the temporal and spatial patterns of expression of a gene in situ can provide a wealth of knowledge regarding the potential functional roles of a gene product. However, such detailed analysis of gene expression patterns represents a great challenge to biologists. Classical approaches such as northern blotting, RNAse protection, PCR assays and western blotting are highly reliable and sensitive means of detecting expression, but these methods completely lack spatial information indicating where the gene is expressed. Spatial information can be obtained by the use of similar approaches such as in situ hybridization and immunohistochemistry on tissue sections or whole tissue preparations. These methods, however, are limited by the availability of robust and reliable probes for the gene of interest as well as the availability of appropriately prepared tissues to probe. Even under optimal conditions, such approaches are not practical when the aim is to undertake an exhaustive screen to discover rare sites of expression in a range of ages.

The use of genetically inserted reporter genes with optimal detection characteristics, most notably the bacterial *LacZ* gene encoding β-galactosidase (β-Gal), in vivo by either targeted or transgenic insertion, allows one to screen a diverse array of tissues and developmental stages rapidly and easily, and to observe domains of expression with extremely high resolution. Coupling of reporter gene insertion with gene targeting and inactivation in mice represents an extremely powerful tool for elucidating gene function, allowing high resolution analysis of domains of expression coupled with the potential loss-of-function phenotypes of the gene of interest. This approach has been used with a great deal of success over the past 10 years in genetargeting, and considerably longer (but without the phenotypic component and with significant limitations) using randomly integrated constructs harboring the reporter gene downstream of the presumed promoter of a gene of interest. We favor the approach of utilizing a rational and standardized construct design that allows a chosen site of integration to be targeted. We will focus our discussion on the use of this approach.

The success of gene expression analysis using reporter genes in mice is highly dependent on a well designed targeting vector. Such designs rely greatly on the ability to place the reporter gene in a precise location within an endogenous locus. Until recently, the construction of such precisely designed vectors was hampered by the limitations of classical molecular biology techniques. However, the advent of the use of bacterial homologous recombination in generating targeting vectors has largely eliminated these difficulties and now allows the execution of practically any vector design with nucleotide precision. We have developed a technology we call "Veloci-Gene" to achieve such goals with incredible success in a very large number of gene targeting projects.

Despite having the ability to minimize unwanted changes that may adversely affect reporter function by manipulating the genome with great precision, factors such as RNA stability and transcriptional and translational controls can also have significant effects on the normal expression of the gene of interest. Engineering the gene of interest by inserting a reporter and deleting and/or adding controlling elements (including the introduction of a non endogenous polyadenylation signal) might result in the reporter gene not being subject to all of the normal levels of control. Therefore, despite the clear advantages of using reporter genes in mice, it is important to bear in mind the parameters of the technology. Thus, it is appropriate to view a reporter gene in mice as most accurately reflecting promoter activity of the gene of interest rather than an ultimate indication of the precise levels of expression of the gene being targeted.

This chapter incorporates the extensive experience accrued from designing and analyzing hundreds of mouse gene-targeted models, in which a variety of reporter genes have been introduced in order to understand the normal or pathological pattern of expression of the gene of interest. This chapter should serve as a guide to users of transgenic and gene targeting technology in the selection of appropriate reporter genes for expression analysis; to provide some information regarding the design of optimal reporter gene constructs; and to provide detailed methods for the optimal detection of reporter genes in situ.

Reporter Genes

Selection of the Appropriate Reporter Gene

Before embarking on generating a mouse reporter knock-in, it is important to consider what the goals of the project are, because these goals can often inform one as to what the best reporter gene will be for a particular application. We will discuss the use of the best characterized reporter genes that have been used successfully in mice. These include *enhanced green florescent protein* (eGFP), placental alkaline phosphatase (PLAP), β-galactosidase (β-Gal), and a variety of derivatives thereof. The relative advantages and disadvantages of each are discussed.

Table 13.1 briefly summarizes the various strengths of the reporter genes we have tested in our high throughput expression-screening laboratory. Subsequent tables will discuss these attributes in greater detail on a reporter-by-reporter basis. We also provide a flow diagram to guide the user in the selection of the appropriate reporter for a given scientific application.

Table 13.1. Comparison of reporter genes with respect to their key features.

	Fluorescent proteins	*PLAP*	*LacZ*	*Nuc-LacZ*	*TM-LacZ*
Sensitivity	Low	Highest	High	Very high	Very high
Penetration of thick tissues	Low	Moderate	Excellent	Excellent	Excellent
Resolution in thick tissues	Low	High	High	Highest	Very high
Cell counting	No	No	No	Yes	No
Cell/process resolution	OK/good	Excellent	OK	No	Good
Viable imaging	Yes	No	No	No	No
Ease of use	Difficult	Less easy	Very easy	Very easy	Very easy

Fluorescent proteins

An ever-expanding range of fluorescent proteins is available for potential use as expression reporters. One of the most widely used is eGFP. There are a great many reasons for choosing to work with eGFP as a reporter, the principal one being the ability to visualize the reporter in the tissues of living mice. Another is that eGFP has been used extensively as a fusion protein in mice with good success. However, if these are not critical aspects of the gene targeting experiment, one should probably consider other reporter genes for their various advantages over eGFP. In contrast to enzymatic reporter genes, eGFP can be visualized directly by using appropriate illumination and filter systems. However, because eGFP is a non-endogenous gene product in mice, it is amenable to detection by immunohistochemistry using anti-GFP antiserum as an alternative means of its detection. There are acceptable anti-sera for use in this application, as has been nicely demonstrated, for example in the GENSAT (*gene expression nervous system atlas*) project. Direct visualization of eGFP and immunohistochemistry each have their own sets of advantages and disadvantages. For example, although using immunohistochemistry to detect eGFP does not take advantage of the simplicity of direct detection, or allow visualization in living tissue, it does permit superior fixation and preservation of tissues, which allows for long-term storage and superior tissue morphology.

Table 13.2. Issues to be considered when working with fluorescent proteins as reporter genes

Resolution in thick tissues. It is extremely difficult to resolve individual cells or their processes in tissues more than 0:5 mm thick due to the limitations of optics, and signal-to-noise issuese GFP can be used to visualize whole metastatic cancers in living mice

Penetration of thick tissue. Reagent penetration is not relevant for detecting eGFP because it is directly visualizedImmunohistochemistry as an alternative means of detection of eGFP, however, is highly subject to tissue penetration issues and is generally limited in use to fairly thin preparations of tissue

The use of immunohistochemistry allows better fixation of the tissue, resulting in the ability to store tissues and to achieve better morphology. It also opens the possibility of amplifying the signal during the process. Despite the clear utility of this type of approach for some applications, it does not take full advantage that reporter genes generally afford. For example, it does not allow the screening of large pieces of tissues, and it adds an expensive and time-consuming element to the process of screening expression patterns

Sensitivity. Compared to other expression reporters, eGFP is not a sensitive mechanism for detecting gene expression

Cell counting. eGFP is generally not the first choice of expression reporter, unless counting of living cells is necessary

Cell/process resolution. eGFP can be a useful tool for tracing neuronal connections in vivo and the dynamic processes involved in kidney development. Because it is a relatively small protein it is possible that it distributes well within a cell, including its processes

Viable imaging. Fluorescent proteins like eGFP are effectively the only way to visualize gene expression in living tissues and animals

Fluorescent proteins are excellent reagents if the goal is to sort cells in a FACS machine. This use becomes all the more powerful when different fluorescent reporters are used to separate different populations from the same tissue sample

Ease of use. Visualization of eGFP requires proper (expensive) microscopic equipment. This also adds an element of inconvenience to the analysis Because fluorescence is frequently diminished by fixation or storage, it requires that tissues be screened shortly after harvest. This can put a significant burden on the researcher to evaluate and document results promptly eGFP is a relatively weak fluorochrome. Therefore, few endogenous promoters will drive expression at sufficiently high levels for eGFP to be easily visible. This is compounded by strong auto-fluorescence of mouse tissues in the range that eGPF fluoresces. This can be addressed, but only by expensive and involved spectral imaging approaches

Other variants. We have had great success using eGFP, but have been less satisfied by the results obtained when CFP (cyan fluorescent protein) and dsRed2 are inserted into an otherwise strongly expressing locus. CFP appears to be an order of magnitude less fluorescent than eGFP, and dsRed2 has been undetectable in a configuration that generated brightly fluorescent mice when eGFP was inserted in an identical manner. We have had success recently using JRed, a novel red fluorescent protein obtained by mutagenesis of Anthomedusae jellyfish chromoprotein, which, although relatively weak in florescence compared to eGFP, has good signal to background characteristics in vivo. In addition, recent success has been reported when using DsRed T3, a new variant of DsRed in mice

---

Fluorescent proteins are generally amenable to fusing with other cellular proteins. Thus, they can be readily targeted to a wide variety of sub-cellular compartments to aid in determining which cell type expresses the gene of interest. This can also lead to a better understanding of cellular activities within that cell. A good example is the use of a histone fusion protein (H2B-eGFP) to visualize the cell nucleus in resting cells and mitotic figures in dividing cells. Another example is the use of membrane-targeted (e.g., by fusion to transmembrane domain-containing sequences or by farnesylation) fluorescent proteins to aid in the visualization of cellular morphology and cellular projections such as *axons* and *filopodia*.

Given that scientists are always searching for fluorescent reporters that can be more readily visualized compared to eGFP, there is a strong drive to discover and enhance naturally occurring fluorescent proteins. Recently, an alternative, yellow fluorescent protein that is faster maturing and brighter than other currently available proteins was reported, raising the possibility of more widespread uses for fluorescent proteins as reporters; however, we have not yet evaluated this protein as a reporter gene in mice.

Placental Alkaline Phosphatase

PLAP is a well-characterized reporter protein that is frequently used in cell-based assays. We have found it to be a reliable and sensitive reporter for revealing gene expression. The histochemical reaction product has a dark-blue/purple color that is easy to see in mice, and is readily combined with counter stains in sections. A distinct advantage of PLAP over other reporters is its high sensitivity.

Table 13.3. Issues to be considered when working with PLAP as a reporter gene

Resolution in thick tissues. The reaction product generated by PLAP is stable and allows tissues to be cleared to improve the visibility of stain. We regularly use glycerol for this purpose, though an alternative superior clearing method using BABB can be used, but is relatively toxic. For this reason we routinely clear in 70% glycerol

Penetration of thick tissues. When intense, the reaction product can create a relatively impermeable barrier to the staining solution, prohibiting visualization of reporter gene expression below the stained surface Providing that the whole structure being stained does not contain PLAP, then the histochemical reaction penetrates tissues reliably

As with fluorescent reporters, good commercial antibodies to PLAP are available, but have the same caveats as for detecting eGFP

Sensitivity. Assays for detecting PLAP are very sensitive

The use of PLAP to reveal gene expression suffers from various drawbacks, the main one being that several tissues (e.g., bone, placenta, intestine) express relatively high levels of endogenous phosphatases. This requires that endogenous activity in these tissues be heat inactivated to diminish this background, degrading tissue morphology in the process. Endogenous alkaline phosphatases can also be inhibited by Levamisole; however, in our experience, this also reduces specific signal without being sufficiently effective in reducing non-specific activity, and therefore is not recommended

Cell counting. Not an optimal reporter, given that the whole cell is stained, not just the nucleus

Cell/process resolution. PLAP is excellent for revealing cell morphology and is particularly highly valued for tracing neuronal processes

PLAP can lead to a slight fuzzy appearance of the reaction product at higher magnifications

Viable imaging. Viable imaging is not possible when using PLAP

Ease of use. PLAP is a more stable enzyme than β-Gal and as such is not as sensitive to short-term storage of tissues prior to staining

The staining procedure requires a heat inactivation step, but is otherwise simple and relatively inexpensive to complete

Unlike β-Gal, the PLAP staining solution can discolor non- expressing tissues if the reaction solution is not changed frequently

As with β-Gal, the staining reaction is light sensitive

LacZ (β-Gal)

The bacterial *LacZ* gene, which encodes β-Gal, has been widely used for many years as a reporter gene. Its use is well characterized in mice and in many ways it is ideally suited for this task. There are various straightforward and standardized protocols for revealing the presence of β-Gal. One of the great advantages of β-Gal is that its presence can be revealed by a simple and relatively cheap reaction in the presence of X-Gal (5-bromo-4-chloro-3- indolyl β-D-glucopyranoside). The reaction generates a blue product that is visually pleasing, stable and easy to detect.

Table 13.4. Issues to be considered when working with LacZ as a reporter gene

---

Resolution in thick tissues. LacZ is our reagent of choice

The histochemical product is stable and is easy to see when tissues have been cleared in glycerol.

LacZ-stained tissues can also be cleared with BABB; however, the signal will also be cleared over a period of a few days

Penetration of thick tissues. When the protocol in this chapter is used, excellent results can be achieved when staining with thick tissues

Sensitivity. β-Gal detection is moderately sensitive, and the standard protocol is sufficient for most endogenous promoters

When increased sensitivity is required, the histochemical reaction can be modified to make it more sensitive

Cell counting. LacZ is not ideal for counting cells as the whole cell body can end up being stained, making cells difficult to distinguish from neighboring cells

Cell/process resolution. This is frequently possible when using LacZ, particularly when very high levels of expression are achieved

It can be improved if LacZ is fused to tau or TM, which results in β-Gal being transported to cell processes such as axons via microtubule binding or to the cell membrane in the case of TM

Viable imaging. LacZ cannot be visualized in living animals

Other reagents [e.g. FDG (fluorescein digalactoside) from Molecular Probes, Eugene, OR] fluoresce when cleaved by β-Gal and can be used in live β-Gal-expressing cells that can be sorted in a FACS machine, though loading cells with the FDG substrate and retaining the resultant signal in the expressing cells can be challenging

Ease of use. Very easy

The histochemical reaction is light sensitive

One of the potential drawbacks to visualizing β-Gal with X- Gal is that one is relying on an enzymatic reaction (cleaving galactose from X-Gal). This means that care should be taken to avoid any steps that would result in protein degradation, including extended fixation and delays in processing, both of which β-Gal is sensitive to

If degradation cannot be avoided, commercially available antibodies can also be used to detect the presence of β-Gal

Other variants. As alluded to above, variants of LacZ created by fusing it to other protein domains are available.

This X-Gal-based assay has been routinely used to screen for expression in young embryos and in histological sections. We have adapted it for high throughput screening of gene expression in whole-mount adult tissues, as described in the protocols section. This novel use of the assay in whole adult tissues allows us to exhaustively screen for the presence of reporter gene expression throughout the entire adult mouse with a high degree of spatial resolution without having to resort to cutting serial sections through extensive sets of tissues. With practice, perfusion and tissue preparation can take as little as 20–30 min per mouse. For most applications, LacZ is the reporter gene of choice due to its ease of use and its ability to be detected with high resolution, even in thick tissue preparations.

TM-LacZ (transmembrane LacZ), NL-LacZ (nuclear localized LacZ) and other LacZ fusions

As with eGFP, it is possible to fuse LacZ with other protein constituents to cause LacZ to be transported to specific compartments within the cell. This approach can be considered, for example, in applications in which it would be advantageous to be able to visualize the membrane surface and/or cellular processes of the expressing cells

(TM-LacZ or Tau LacZ) or if it is desirable to carefully quantify the numbers of expressing cells (NL-LacZ) in the genetically altered mice. When targeting genes with a signal peptide (i.e., secreted and transmembrane-domain-containing genes), it can be highly advantageous to retain the endogenous signal peptide (frequently encoded by exon 1 in such genes), and substitute a TM-LacZ reporter in downstream exons to create a fusion with the endogenous signal sequence. After postranslational processing, this TM-β-Gal protein will be deposited below the cell surface. Targeting the gene in this way allows one to avoid targeting potential regulatory sequences in the vicinity of the initiating codon of the gene of interest. Because this simplifies the design of a targeting vector, avoids the pitfalls of deleting potential regulatory sequences, and retains all of the advantages of using LacZ as a preferred reporter gene, this is our selection of choice when targeting secreted and transmembrane-domain-containing genes. Table 13.5 gives examples of when the use of different LacZ fusions might be advantageous.

Table 13.5. Relative advantages to using LacZ fusions

NL-LacZ. It is frequently difficult to resolve individual cells because the LacZ protein diffuses to fill much of the cell. However, by fusing LacZ to a nuclear localizing signal, the LacZ product is sequestered to the nucleus, thus overcoming this problem

Because it is discreetly localized in the nucleus, NL-LacZ allows one to readily count and quantify numbers of expressing cells

NL-LacZ is generally more easily detected compared to normal LacZ, possibly due to the concentration effect of the β-Gal enzymatic activity within the confines of the nucleus, as well as the fact that the resulting signal is more discretely localized and concentrated

Because the nucleus of the expressing cell is all that is visualized, one loses the important advantages of seeing cellular shapes - often a critical aid in positively identifying the cell type expressing β-Gal

TM-LacZ. TM-LacZ is a good reagent for creating knock-ins into signal peptide-containing genes such as secreted and transmembrane proteins

This allows insertion of the reporter gene in exons downstream of the signal peptide-encoding exons and avoids the potential complications and compromises in gene expression that may occur when a reporter and selection cassette are integrated near the promoter of a gene, or when integration inadvertently disrupts regulatory sequences in the first intron of a gene

In contrast to normal LacZ, TM-LacZ fusions generally distribute over the surface of the expressing cell, which gives the staining a different quality of appearance, which sometimes aids in positively identifying the expressing cell type

TM-LacZ fusions generally are more sensitive and readily detected compared to normal LacZ due to concentration of β-Gal at the cell membrane

Tau-LacZ. Tau is a protein that is associated with the cell scaffold

Fusion of LacZ with tau results in β-Gal being associated with the cell's microtubules

Neuronal projections and other cellular processes can be dramatically revealed by using this LacZ fusion

Reporter Constructs

Position Effects

Given the flexibility, modular design, and throughput of the VelociGene process, we have been able to test the same reporter gene in various positions within a gene of interest. In several loci, we have found that subtly changing the insertion point relative to the endogenous promoter can have significant effects on the strength of the reporter signal and fidelity of the expression pattern. Since transcription regulatory sequences often reside within the first intron, when possible, we have found it to be good practice to insert the TM-LacZ reporter cassette into the second exon to generate a transmembrane fusion reporter. Because regulatory sequences can reside anywhere in a gene of interest it is valuable to compare genomic sequences from multiple species (e.g., mouse versus human) as a crude means of elucidating potential regulatory elements in non-coding regions. Where possible, one should avoid deletion of regions conserved across species. Often, however, compromises regarding the final deletion must be made to balance the desire to obliterate gene function with the desire to achieve faithful reporter gene expression. These decisions must be made on a case-by-case basis. It is also worthwhile mentioning that the proximity of the promoter and selection cassette in your targeting vector can have unwanted influences on the faithful expression of your reporter gene. Such effects should also be mitigated by placing the insertion away from the endogenous promoter, but can also be amended if the selection cassette has been flanked by loxP sites, allowing removal of the cassette by excision using Cre recombinase, thus we recommend this practice.

Multiple transgenes from the same promoter

Although the use of internal ribosome entry site (IRES)-containing cassettes is quite widespread, we have found that the levels of the two trans- genes can be rather unpredictable, with the first transgene frequently being expressed at a much higher level than the transgene following the IRES sequence. Even when a bicistronic cassette has been highly optimized, it is not likely to achieve relatively high levels of expression of either trans- gene, much less both of them. For these reasons, we have generally avoided the use of bicistronic approaches for revealing gene expression patterns in mice, and do not recommend them for general use.

PROTOCOLS

This section contains detailed methods for the detection of the reporter genes described above, for both whole-mount and sectioned embryos and adult tissues. When appropriate, we also describe dissection procedures in detail as well as methods to fashion helpful tools.

Silicone Plates

There are many occasions when it is useful to immobilize tissues, either during particularly delicate or challenging dissections, or when photo- documenting results. To accomplish this, coat glass Petri dishes with a layer of silicone elastomer, and pin specimens down on this substrate using fine dissecting pins. Such a substrate is durable and clear, and allows transillumination of specimens during dissection, observation and photo-documentation. It is also sometimes useful to dissect or photograph tissues on a dark background. Adding activated charcoal to the unpolymerized silicone solution will achieve this effect. The use of silicone elastomer substrates has the added benefit of minimizing damage to delicate instruments during dissection. We generally have both clear and black plates available at all times.

Use 10 cm and 15 cm diameter glass Petri dishes coated with 5 mm Sylgard. For plates with a black background, add enough activated charcoal for the unpolymerized solution to turn black. The amount will be in the order of 5% of the total volume. When the solution sets it frequently becomes lighter, so it is better to add more charcoal, than less. Best polymerization is achieved by incubating the dishes overnight at 37°C.

Dissection of Embryos for Whole-mount Staining for β-Gal or PLAP visualization

General comments

1. Younger embryos (less than E12.5) generally need little dissection beyond removal from the uterus and yolk sac. Older embryos require

varying degrees of sub-dissection to ensure that tissues are evenly stained.

2. Since this method relies on the enzymatic properties of β-Gal or PLAP, it is important to avoid over-fixing or storing embryos prior to staining. Also, it is best to keep all reagents and tissues on wet ice throughout the dissection.
3. Sacrifice pregnant dam according to local animal use policies.
4. If embryos are to be genotyped, clean dissection tools before each embryo to avoid cross-contamination of the next sample.
5. Use Petri dishes with a base of black silicone to aid in visualization, and so that tissues can be pinned out if the embryos need dissecting.
6. All incubations take place on rockers to ensure that the tissues are gently agitated. We use a cycle rate of approximately 15–30 agitations per minute.

Materials required

1. 50 ml centrifuge tubes
2. 12- or 24-well tissue culture plates (depending on the age/size of the embryo)
3. 25 ml glass scintillation vials
4. dissection instruments
5. Tubes for collecting tissues for genotyping
6. PBS (pH 8)
7. Freshly made 4% paraformaldehyde
8. DNA lysis buffer (if needed for genotyping)

Dissection

1. Remove uterus and keep on ice in PBS.
2. Cut open uterus along length on side. Remove embryos, with yolk sac and placenta intact.
3. Extract embryo from yolk sac. Let embryo bleed out for a while in the PBS (hemoglobin inhibits the staining reaction and obscures positive staining in the vasculature). Rinse with PBS. Keep embryos in PBS on ice.
4. If embryos are to be genotyped, keep yolk sac or cut off tail and place in DNA lysis buffer in a 96-well plate overnight at 55°C. Embryos will have to be stained separately.
5. If embryos are E12.5 or younger, place in fixative. If embryos are E13.5 or older, dissect as described in step 6. E18.5 or older mice should be anesthetized (we use a mix of Ketamine:Xylazine

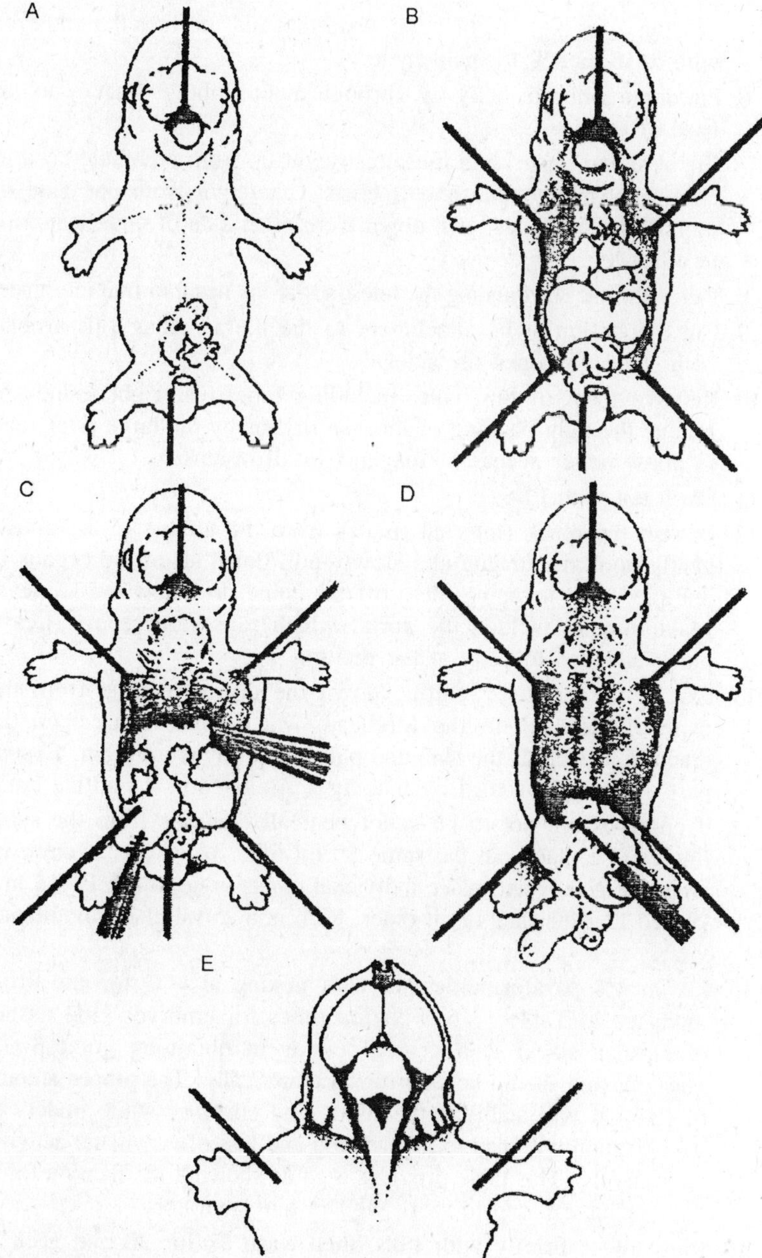

Fig. 13.1. A-E Embryo dissection guide.

120 mg:5 mg/kg). After being anaesthetized, perfuse the embryos with 5–10 ml 4% formaldehyde.

6. Pin down embryo, belly up, through mouth (above tongue) and at base of tail.
7. Cut skin and underlying muscle straight up from umbilical cord to chin, exposing tongue and trachea. Cut down from one side of umbilical cord to leg. Cut down from other side of umbilical cord to other leg.
8. Pierce the sac surrounding the intestines at the naval to free intestines.
9. Cut diaphragm at its attachment to the thorax along ribs around both sides. Pin open the sides.
10. Remove most of the liver, including lobe over right kidney to relieve the tight packing of internal organs by the large liver, and to allow better access of reagents to all organs.
11. Flush out with PBS.
12. Dissect the pluck (internal tissues from the tongue to the anus): gently hook the tongue and slowly pull down all of the organs in one piece, by scraping them off the spine, to below the kidneys. Make sure to include the aorta, which runs along spine. Leave pluck attached to body at the rectum.
13. Expose the brain by cutting down the dorsal midline from the nape of the neck to the forehead. Make sure to cut open the cranium as well as the skin and pull both away from brain. Expose part of the spinal cord by making a similar dorsal midline cut.
14. If embryos are not to be genotyped, all embryos from the same line can be placed in the same 50 ml tube. However, if embryos are to be genotyped, place individual embryos up to age E13.5 in a labeled 12-well plate or, if older, each in a 25 ml glass scintillation vial.
15. Fix in 4% paraformaldehyde with mixing at 4°C for the times indicated in Table 13.6. Fixation times for embryos (and tissues of similar sizes) is a critical factor in obtaining good β-Gal reactions and should be determined empirically. The proper amount of fixation will stabilize the tissue and enzyme, while under- or over-fixation will lead to degradation and loss of enzymatic activity, respectively. This table provides a guide showing the fixation times that we have found to work well in our laboratory.
16. Rinse twice briefly with PBS, then wash 3x for 20 min each in large volumes of PBS at 4°C with agitation (paraformaldehyde inhibits LacZ staining).

Table 13.6. Suggested fixation times for embryos of varying ages

Embryo age	Fix time (min) 4°C
E8.5–E11.5	15 min
E12.5–E14.5	30 min
E15.5–E17.5	60 min

Whole-mount Staining of Embryos for LacZ

Examples of whole-mount stained embryos of various ages revealing a number of interesting patterns of expression in a variety of tissues and regions of the embryo.

Materials required

1. PBS (pH 8.0)
2. Rocking platform shakers (at 4°C)
3. LacZ staining solution
4. 50% glycerol
5. 70% glycerol
6. 4% paraformaldehyde

Staining method

1. Dissect and fix embryos as described above.
2. Incubate embryos in LacZ staining solution for up to 48 h in the dark at 4°C.
3. Rinse briefly in cold PBS and then wash in cold PBS for 15 min.
4. Postfix in 4% paraformaldehyde at 4°C overnight on the rocker.
5. Incubate in 50% glycerol on a rocker overnight at 4°C, then clear in 70% glycerol.
6. Final storage at room temperature in 70% glycerol.

Whole-mount PLAP Staining of Embryos

Materials required

1. Dissection instruments
2. Heated water bath
3. 25 ml glass scintillation vials
4. 50 ml centrifuge tubes
5. BCIP solution (Roche)
6. NBT solution (Roche)
7. PBS (pH 7.4)
8. Fresh 4% paraformaldehyde in PBS

9. NTMT buffer
10. 50% glycerol
11. 70% glycerol

Dissection and preparation for staining

1. Pre-heat the water bath to 75°C.
2. Follow steps described above
3. Transfer embryos in PBS to individual 25 ml glass scintillation vials.
4. To inactivate endogenous phosphatases, heat treat the embryos in PBS for 30 min in the water bath, agitating gently every 10 min.
5. Transfer vials to ice to cool, and wash the embryos twice in PBS for 5 min each. If necessary the samples can be stored at 4°C overnight at this point.
6. Transfer samples to 50 ml centrifuge tubes and wash three times for 20 min with cold NTMT buffer.
7. Stain the samples in NTMT buffer with 1 μl BCIP and 1 μl NBT per milliliter at 4°C on a rocker in the dark.
8. To stop the reaction, wash embryos in PBS and then place embryos in 4% paraformaldehyde overnight.
9. Transfer the embryos to 50% glycerol overnight before storing them in 70% glycerol solution.

   To minimize non-specific staining:

(a) Change to fresh staining solution as soon as there is a purple tinge to the solution

(b) Avoid exposing the staining solution to light

(c) Keep the staining reaction and solutions at 4°C.

Dissection of Adult Tissue

Whole adult animals can be subjected to a modified version of the whole- mount analysis described above for E15.5 embryos. This technique can be highly valuable for obtaining an exhaustive survey of virtually the entire animal to determine if the reporter gene is expressed. In this assay, the organs are freed from their tight associations with other tissues, and tissues of thickness greater than approximately 2 mm are sliced at intervals to allow access of reagents. We generally employ this adult whole-mount procedure as a screening process to determine all possible sites of expression of β-Gal in the adult, and use this information to inform us as to how to proceed with high resolution analysis employing thin sections of target tissues.

Examples of data from whole-mount adult tissues reveal a variety of the high quality of data that can be readily obtained from this crude technique.

Materials required

1. Perfusion pump or 50 ml syringe
2. 25G syringe needles
3. 125 ml amber/brown centrifuge bottles
4. 50 ml centrifuge tubes
5. Rocking platform shakers
6. Dissection instruments
7. Tubes for collecting tissues for genotyping
8. PBS (pH 8)
9. Freshly made 4% paraformaldehyde in PBS
10. DNA lysis buffer (if genotyping mice)

Perfusion

Note: Tissue samples for northern/Southern blot and genotyping or blood samples should be collected prior to perfusion of the animal.

1. Anesthetize the mouse according to local animal use guidelines.
2. Once the mouse is clearly anesthetized (check by pinching toe and/or by eliciting a blink response), cut the skin overlying the rib cage and open the abdominal cavity by cutting the abdominal wall at the edge of the rib cage. Open the chest cavity by separating the rib cage from the diaphragm. Be careful to not damage any organs below, especially the liver, lungs and heart, which may lead to poor perfusion.
3. Cut the right atrium and perfuse through the left ventricle with cold 4% paraformaldehyde using the perfusion pump. This should take 20 min per mouse using a flow rate set at 3 ml/min.

Dissection

Note: While each organ of interest can be carefully dissected and removed from its associated tissues to be processed, the following procedure is routinely performed in our lab to make the process as rapid and thorough as possible. This method has the added advantage of keeping tissues in their normal bodily context, which can aid in identifying reporter gene expressing tissues and cells.

1. Prepare a labeled 125 ml amber bottle with 50 ml cold PBS for each animal and put it on ice. It will serve as container for tissue collection and future tissue processing.

2. Remove the skin from the surface of the rib cage. Dissect away and keep the ventral half of the rib cage containing the sternum and both cartilaginous and bony sections of rib.
3. Remove right ear at its base and carefully pull apart the two opposing layers of skin to expose the cartilage and muscle between them to the staining solution.
4. Remove brain from skull, then carefully slice brain with a razor along the midline. Cut brain into crude 2 mm thick slabs to allow access of reagents to various parts of the brain.
5. Open the abdomen by making two lateral incisions. Keep the freed abdominal muscle tissue separated from the overlying skin. Collect two of the abdominal mammary glands, slicing one of them in half using a razor blade.
6. Dissect all tissues from the tongue to end of the colon and all of the associated tissue and viscera. Do this by gently hooking the tongue and slowly pulling down all of the organs in one piece, by scraping/severing them from the interior surface of the dorsal body wall and spine. Make sure to include the thoracic and abdominal aorta, which runs along the spine. Also gently hook the genital area and pull up all the organs in one piece, again by scraping/severing them from the interior surface of the dorsal body wall and spine. Avoid any damage to the intestine, whose contents can foul the LacZ histochemical reaction. Remove the whole collection of tissues from the rest of the animal.
7. To allow better penetration of the staining solution, the tongue, heart, lungs, liver, spleen and kidneys should have multiple small razor cuts along the midline. We find it most convenient to fall short of cutting completely through the organ to ensure that the tissues remain connected and can be later viewed in context following staining.
8. Cut off the remaining skull and split it along the midline with a razor blade.
9. Remove the brown fat from between the shoulder blades.
10. Keep a piece of the skin from the back.
11. Remove the spinal cord/vertebrae and associated muscle, bone and other tissues and remove surrounding tissue from the anterior portion of this to expose about 5 mm of spinal cord.
12. Remove the hind limb and pull the skin off. Slit the paw open with a razor all the way to the tip of the digit, ideally splitting the footpad in half.

13. Fix all collected tissues in 4% paraformaldehyde at 4°C for 30 min on a rocker.
14. Rinse twice briefly with PBS.
15. Wash the tissues three times for 20 min each in PBS at 4°C (paraformaldehyde inhibits LacZ staining).

Preparing Embryos and Adult Tissues for Cryo-Sectioning

Following analysis of results from the above whole-mount procedures, target tissues expressing the reporter gene can be greatly narrowed, and can then be examined with the following high resolution methods.

High resolution expression analysis using the reporter genes described in this chapter can be achieved by creating sections of target tissues of varying thickness and using varying methods. Most commonly, sections are obtained through the use of one of three common methods and devices. One method utilizes a vibrating blade microtome, which is suitable for use on soft and uniform pieces of fresh, unfrozen tissues to generate fairly thick, free-floating sections (generally ranging from 30 to 500 μm in thickness). A second method utilizes a sliding microtome, which is also suitable for soft and uniform tissues that are cut when frozen to create free floating sections of intermediate thickness (generally ranging from 40 to 100 μm). Finally, another method utilizes a cryostat, which is capable of cutting a whole range of tissues, including those containing bone, and which can create sections in the thin-to-moderately thick range (generally 5–40 μm), which are generally applied directly to microscope slides while still frozen. The method used to create sections of tissue is to some degree a matter of personal preference and/or is dependent on available sectioning equipment. We use all three techniques, depending on the goals of our experiments, but as a matter of routine we employ a cryostat to create sections. We discuss in detail only the use of the cryostat as a method of performing high resolution analysis in this chapter.

Materials required

1. Dissection equipment
2. 25 ml glass scintillation vials (for embryos)
3. 125 ml centrifuge bottles (for adult mice)
4. OCT (TissueTek)
5. Embedding molds (size appropriate to tissue to be cut)
6. 2-Methylbutane (isopotane)
7. Dry ice

8. Lint-free tissues
9. PBS (pH 8.0)
10. Fresh 4% paraformaldehyde in PBS (pH 8.0)
11. 15% sucrose (w/v) in PBS (pH 8.0)
12. 30% sucrose (w/v) in PBS (pH 8.0)

Dissection

1. Follow step 1 through 4 as described above.
2. Fix un-eviscerated embryos or dissected tissues from adults in 4% paraformaldehyde for 30 min with agitation at 4°C. Do not make extra cuts in adult tissue blocks as this will make sectioning more difficult. Embryos of E15.5 and older have to be slit open along the right side of the abdomen, thorax and head to allow complete fixation of the internal organs.
3. Rinse tissues twice briefly with PBS and then wash three times for 20 min each with PBS.
4. Equilibrate in 15% sucrose until tissues sink to bottom of vial/tube (overnight) at 4°C and subsequently in 30% sucrose overnight at 4°C.

Embedding

1. Choose convenient mold size. The mold should be large enough to ensure that the tissues are completely submersed in OCT.
2. Remove excess sucrose carefully with a lint-free tissue.
3. Tissues should be embedded according to orientation required. We routinely cut sagittal sections of embryos. We label the outside of the mold to ensure that we can orient the block to the knife without difficulty (OCT becomes opaque when it freezes).
4. Cover tissue in OCT taking care to avoid introducing bubbles. Bubbles will mean that the tissues are not supported evenly in the frozen OCT, resulting in sections that are distorted and uneven.
5. Place mold in dry-ice-chilled 2-methylbutane until completely frozen.
6. The frozen blocks can be stored short-term on dry ice or long-term at –80°C.

Cryo-sectioning

Materials required

1. Cryostat
2. OCT (TissueTek)
3. Acid alcohol

4. Poly-L-lysine solution
5. Microscope slides
6. Microscope coverslips
7. Coverslipping medium
8. Graded alcohols for dehydrating sections prior to coverslipping
9. Xylene or xylene substitute for clearing prior to coverslipping

Slide preparation

1. Clean microscope slides with acid alcohol.
2. Place a rack of clean slides for 5 min in 1:10 diluted poly-L-lysine solution at room temperature.
3. Dry slides for 1 h at 60°C.

An alternative to coating slides with poly-L-lysine is to use charged slides available from various manufacturers, such as SuperPlus slides from VWR. Although they provide significant time savings, we find that they do not function as well as poly-L-lysine coated slides.

Another option is to use the CryoJane Tape Transfer System developed by Instrumedics. This system uses a two-step process for attaching cryostat sections to the microscope slide. The first involves applying a tape to the tissue block face. The section is then cut and comes away attached to the transfer tape. Tape-backed sections are applied to a microscope slide coated with a UV-polymerizable adhesive. The adhesive is activated on the slide with a UV pulse. The transfer tape is then removed and the tissue remains attached to the slide. A distinct advantage of the tape transfer system is that almost completely distortion-free frozen sections can be obtained, even from very large specimens.

We routinely use this system when sectioning whole embryos and many other tissues (especially those with bone), as the sections are free from the normal distortion encountered with typical cryostat sections, and tissues containing bone and cartilage can be sectioned without resorting to decalcification steps.

Sectioning

We regularly cut 20 μm sections to stain for the presence of β-Gal. We generally prepare a parallel set of sections cut at 10 μm to examine gross morphology through the use of standard histological stains such as Hemotoxylin and Eosin. When sections of varying thickness are collected in an alternating series, be aware of the fact that many cryostats do not cut a uniformly thick section for the first section after the cutting thickness is changed. This means that a section sometimes needs to be discarded after the cutting thickness has been changed.

Once sections have been attached to the slide, it is best to allow them to air-dry for a few minutes at room temperature before storing them at –80°C.

LacZ staining on slides

Note that the histochemical reaction for β-Gal is light sensitive.

1. Retrieve the slides to be stained from –80°C storage.
2. Let the slides to come to room temperature and dry for 30 min at room temperature to increase adhesion to the slides. Do not allow moisture to condense on slides.
3. Stain overnight at 37°C in LacZ staining solution, followed by several rinses in PBS and post fixation in 4% paraformaldehyde for 1 h at 4°C, followed by a mild neutral red or eosin counter stain.

Coverslipping

1. Dehydrate the sections in graded alcohols and place in Xylene substitute for no more than 5 min.
2. Coverslip the slides in a ventilated hood.

Whole-mount Adult LacZ Staining

It is a good idea to include both positive and negative controls (for example, from a wild type and a previously characterized transgenic animal that you are certain to have β-Gal activity) when staining, especially when working with a new project/protocol. This will help to prevent being misled by false positive staining from endogenous galactosidase activity. Another useful indicator as to whether the staining protocol worked is the intestinal contents of adult mice. However, where possible, it is always best to include a positive control specimen.

1. Incubate in LacZ staining solution at 4°C with gentle agitation for up to 48 h. Generally, there seems little to be gained in staining past 48 h. Alternatively, shorter incubations at room temperature or 37°C can be carried out. Although higher incubation temperatures accelerate the development of the reaction product, they have the disadvantages of increasing non-specific staining in whole-mounts and also, importantly, limiting the depth of penetration of the reaction, allowing visualization primarily of superficial staining. For these reasons we routinely develop the stain at 4°C.

2. Rinse in cold PBS and wash in cold PBS for 15 min.
3. Postfix in paraformaldehyde at 4°C overnight on a rocker.
4. Clear with 50% glycerol on a rocker overnight at 4°C.
5. Final clearing and storage in 70% glycerol at room temperature.

Common sites of non-specific staining

Non-specific staining due to endogenous galactosidase activity, most commonly encountered when evaluating β-Gal activity in whole-mounts (especially with prolonged staining times and temperatures above 4°C and/or when staining at low pH), can be misleading. Being aware of these problematic tissues, and staining negative control tissues from age- and sex-matched specimens prepared in parallel are the best defense against being misled when finding staining in them. These tissues include nasal sinuses, lachrymal glands, salivary glands (especially strong staining in males), stomach (pyloric half), intestinal contents, mesenteric lymph nodes, male reproductive organs (testes, epididymis, vas deferens, coagulation glands).

In addition, when the intestine, or its contents, stain very strongly, blue colored fluids can sometimes fill lymphatic vessels, particularly surrounding the gut and in the mesentery, and give the impression of staining in lymphatic vessels. Such false positive staining in closed structures can be identified by the ability to move or drain the apparent stain.

Enhancements to the Standard LacZ Staining Protocol

If the promoter driving the LacZ gene is relatively weak, it is possible to modify the staining solution and replace the ferric and ferrous cyanide with NBT (see recipe at the end of this chapter). This increases the sensitivity of the staining solution by approximately 5- to 10-fold. However, if over incubated, non-targeted tissues can appear to be stained. Our experience is that sections stained at room temperature should not be incubated for longer than 2 h. We have found this enhancement method to be very useful for staining whole embryos up to E15.5. In this case, it is not recommended that embryos be stained beyond 18 h.

We have found that this NBT-containing staining solution brings the sensitivity of the stain close to that for detecting PLAP, which is the most sensitive of reporter genes. However, we have not completed side-by-side comparisons using identical promoters. In addition, like PLAP staining, the NBT/LacZ method results in a more stable deposit, resulting in staining that is more resilient when cleared with BABB.

Stock Solutions

PBS

1. Phosphate-buffered saline (PBS) from 10x stock solution
2. Adjust to pH 8.0 with sodium hydroxide

4% Paraformaldehyde

1. 4% paraformaldehyde solution in PBS, pH 8.0 (made fresh each day, kept ice cold once pH has been adjusted)

Note that paraformaldehyde is toxic, carcinogenic and teratogenic. Ensure that an effective fume hood is used along with personal protective equipment.

NTMT buffer

1. 100 mM NaCl
2. 100 mM Tris pH 9.5
3. 50 mM $MgCl_2$
4. 0.1% Tween-20
5. In distilled water

X-Gal stock

1. 4% (40 mg/ml) in dimethylformamide (DMF) in glass container, protected from light.
2. Store at –20°C

LacZ staining solution

1. 2 mM mM $MgCl_2$
2. 0.01% deoxycholic acid
3. 0.02% IGEPAL CA-630
4. 0.1% (1 mg/ml) X-Gal in DMF
5. 5 mM potassium ferrocyanide (from 100 mM stock in amber bottle)
6. 5 mM potassium ferricyanide (from 100 mM stock in amber bottle) in PBS (pH 8.0)

Alternative (more sensitive) LacZ staining solution

1. 2 mM $MgCl_2$
2. 0.01% deoxycholic acid
3. 0.02% IGEPAL CA630
4. 0.1% (1 mg/ml) X-Gal in DMF
5. 3 μl NBT solution (Roche) per 50 ml
6. in PBS (pH 8.0)

50% Glycerol

1. 50% Glycerol in PBS (pH 7.4)

70% Glycerol

1. 70% Glycerol in PBS (pH 7.4)
2. 0.01% Sodium azide

BABB clearing agent

1. 2 parts benzyl alcohol (v/v)
2. 1 part benzyl benzoate (v/v)

Note: specimens must be dehydrated in a methanol series (25%, 50%, 75%, 95% in PBS and twice in 100% methanol) prior to equilibration with BABB. Insufficient dehydration prior to clearing in BABB will result in the tissue not being properly cleared.

DNA lysis buffer (for 500 ml)

1. 0:1 M Tris HCl pH 7.6
2. 5 mM EDTA
3. 0.2% SDS
4. 0:2 M sodium chloride
   (a) Directly prior to usage, add 100 μl Proteinase K per 5 ml lysis buffer.
   (b) Incubate samples overnight at 55°C prior to DNA extraction and genotyping.

INDEX